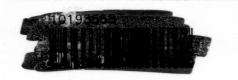

Walking into Darkness

The Experience of Spinal Cord Injury

WALKING INTO DARKNESS

The Experience of Spinal Cord Injury

**M. Oliver*, G. Zarb*, J. Silver†,
M. Moore* and V. Salisbury†**

*School of Education Studies, Thames Polytechnic, London
and
†The National Spinal Injuries Centre, Stoke Mandeville Hospital,
Aylesbury, Bucks.

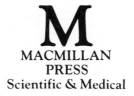

**MACMILLAN
PRESS
Scientific & Medical**

First published 1988

Published by
THE MACMILLAN PRESS LTD
Houndmills, Basingstoke, Hampshire RG21 2XS
and London
Companies and representatives
throughout the world

Distributed in North America by
SHERIDAN HOUSE PUBLISHERS
145 Palisade St, Dobbs Ferry, NY 10522

Typesetting by Footnote Graphics, Warminster, Wilts.

Printed in Great Britain by
The Camelot Press Ltd.
Southampton.

British Library Cataloguing in Publication Data
Walking into darkness.
1. Spinal cord injury victims. Rehabilitation
I. Oliver, M.
613.9'6'08808166
IBSN 0–333–44360–8
ISBN 0–333–44361–6 Pbk

Contents

Preface

For many years, the onset of disability has been viewed as a personal tragedy, and consequently the disabled person has been seen as a victim of such an unfortunate happening. Spinal cord injury has often been seen in such terms: the sudden nature of its occurrence—as the result of a road accident, a fall or a sporting injury—rendering someone who was previously fully fit and well, completely paralysed. The physical consequences of such a happening are best described in the words of Sir Ludwig Guttmann, pioneer in the development of a spinal injury service in the United Kingdom:

> It must be remembered that the spinal cord, that big nerve trunk within the vertebral column, is one of the most important organs in animals and man. For it is the main mediator of all impulses from and to the brain. For instance, any volitional isolated muscle movement initiated from the brain is only possible if the spinal cord is intact, and vice versa—all forms of sensory impulses originating from the skin, muscles, joints and internal organs have to travel through the spinal cord to be consciously appreciated. Moreover, in addition to these vital functions, the cord contains in itself nerve centres for controlling bladder, bowel, sexual and respiratory functions.
>
> Therefore, if the spinal cord is severed or crushed—by a knife, bullet, vascular catastrophe (thrombosis) or a fracture of the spine at any level—this immediately results in a paralysis below the level of the injury, with loss of most essential functions. This involves all voluntary motor functions, appreciation of all forms of sensation, and results in loss of posture and control of bladder and bowels. Sexual function in men is abolished. Women lose sexual sensation but can have intercourse and still conceive. The higher up the spine the level of the injury the more parts of the body are cut off. In injuries of the cervical cord, the respiratory function as well as the blood circulation are greatly impaired, especially in very high cervical lesions, the involvement of the blood circulation leading also to a reduction of the tone of all tissues, especially skin and muscles. This in turn results in a lowering of their resistance to pressure, which is one of the most important causes of the development of pressure sores. All forms of sensation are cut off and the patient does not feel the

discomfort of pressure, such as non-paralysed people do in the form, let us say, of pins and needles.

The victims of war, road, industrial and sporting accidents did not establish a social problem in the past, as their life expectancy was very short, two to three years at the utmost as a rule. Complications such as sepsis from ascending infection of the bladder into the kidneys, and pressure sores, were considered inevitable. Therefore, any attempt to restore such a person to his or her former social activities seemed to be out of the question, and the view generally held was the sooner they died the better for all concerned.

(quoted in Goodman, 1986:96–7)

Given this description, it is not surprising that spinal cord injury is seen as a catastrophic event in someone's life. However, largely as a result of the work of Sir Ludwig Guttmann at Stoke Mandeville Hospital, attitudes to recovery and rehabilitation, and a new approach to spinal cord injury, emerged:

The basic principle of this new philosophy was to provide a comprehensive paraplegia and tetraplegia service to rescue these men, women and children from the human scrapheap and return most of them, in spite of permanent, profound disability—by clinical measures and psychological readjustment—to a life worth living, as useful and respected citizens in the community.

(quoted in Goodman, 1986:101)

Partly as a result of this new approach, many people with spinal cord injury emerged from Stoke Mandeville, and later other hospitals, keen and eager to rebuild their lives or continue their existing ones with the least possible disruption. Not all, of course, made it, but many did and reappeared in society, working, marrying, enjoying a whole range of leisure pursuits and sporting activities, thereby challenging the stereotype of spinal cord injury as a personal tragedy.

The purpose of this book, therefore, is to describe the lives of people with spinal cord injury: to look at what happened to them at the time of their injury, on discharge from the spinal unit and at the time of the interview. Seventy-seven male ex-patients from Stoke Mandeville who had been disabled for between 2 and 15 years were traced and interviewed. The material from the interviews is presented in chronological order, tracing the 'disability career' of those interviewed.

This is not the first study to use the idea of a 'disability career' as a means of providing a chronological or temporal ordering of the data to be presented (Goffman, 1961; Safilios-Rothschild, 1970; Blaxter, 1980). Carver sets out the rationale for such an approach:

A career in disability refers to the course or progress through life of any disabled person insofar as he encounters problems or handicapping conditions related in any way to his disabilities. A person's progress may be affected ... in practical ways and/or in the ways he thinks about himself or others. This concept of career is a broadly comprehensive one and implies that the individual is actively and repeatedly involved in the definition of his own problems and in the search for solutions, and, like any other career, it will comprise a succession of interactions with his environment, both physical and social.

(Carver, 1982:90)

These interactions, at the points in time already mentioned, are described in the words of the people with spinal injuries themselves, giving a sense of authenticity to the disability career.

The first chapter provides a brief history of the medical treatment and rehabilitation of people with a spinal injury, along with an outline of the medical consequences of such an injury and a description of the kinds of treatment facilities available in the United Kingdom. This discussion is located within the context of changing ideas of what are appropriate services for people with a spinal injury and historical changes in the patterns of community support. The second chapter then provides a conceptual framework for the study, seeing spinal cord injury as a 'significant life event' rather than a personal tragedy, and the operationalisation of the concept of social adjustment is also discussed. A short account of the development of the study is provided, together with a description of the methods used to collect the data. Finally, a brief description of some of the characteristics of the people interviewed is presented.

The next three chapters utilise the concept of the career. Chapter 3 focuses on the medical consequences of spinal injury, looking at the nature of the accident, immediate post-accident treatment at both general and specialist hospitals, the rehabilitation process and the medical problems that may arise after discharge and for the rest of the person's life. Chapter 4 then moves away from the immediate medical and physical impact of spinal injury, and focuses on the impact on the injured person and his family. The concept of social adjustment is crucial here, and it is suggested that personal and family responses to spinal injury can only be understood in the light of a whole range of personal, social and economic factors, and not simply as a function of the extent of residual disability. Chapter 5 then broadens out the discussion and looks at the effects that spinal injury has on interpersonal relationships, and the restrictions that it may create for leisure and the pursuit of various hobbies and interests, as well as examining the issues of personal mobility and public transport.

Social adjustment and a successful career in disability are not, however, solely dependent on medical and interpersonal factors: a range of external factors, such as the availability of suitable housing, the prospects of keeping or finding a job and the kind of income support that is available, are also critical. Chapter 6 is pivotal in relation to these issues, for it looks at the roles of various professionals, both within the hospital and in the community. It suggests that while these professionals should provide access to the range of support services, information and benefits available to people with a spinal injury, in practice these roles are inadequately fulfilled.

The next three chapters, therefore, look at the services available. Returning to the concept of disability career, Chapter 7 examines the range of accommodation available, the process of adapting existing properties for someone confined to a wheelchair, and the issue of personal choice about where to live and, indeed, with whom to live. Chapter 8 discusses the effects that spinal injury has on the prospects of keeping an existing job or finding an alternative one, on the capacities and capabilities of those so injured, and on the desire, or otherwise, to resume work. Chapter 9 then describes the financial circumstances of our interviewees and their families, the nature of financial hardships that some of them suffer, and the whole issue of compensation and disability income.

The final chapter then attempts to pull together the many themes that have been raised throughout the book. It summarises the key issues that have arisen; it considers and suggests improvements in the planning and delivery of services, both hospital- and community-based, and it argues that there is urgent need for action by all concerned if the 'disability career' of those with a spinal injury is to be significantly improved.

London and Aylesbury, 1988
M. O.
G. Z.
J. S.
M. M.
V. S.

Acknowledgements

We are grateful to the King Edward's Hospital Fund for London and the Jules Thorn Trust, who funded the research on which this book is based. The Spinal Injuries Association and the National Spinal Injuries Centre at Stoke Mandeville Hospital provided additional funds, and we are also grateful for their encouragement and support.

Without the help of two people in particular, this book might never have seen the light of day. Gill Creek was responsible for the coding and analysis of our statistical data and, hence, for giving our work a coherence it might not otherwise have had. Cathy Lewington typed the manuscript with such speed and efficiency that she was able to keep us supplied with tea when we needed it most, and it is thanks to her that the manuscript was not as late as it would otherwise have been.

Most of all, we owe an enormous debt of gratitude to those people with spinal injuries who allowed us to intrude on their lives and invade their privacy. Without them, there would have been no book, although, of course, any shortcomings in the final product are ours, not theirs.

CHAPTER 1

Spinal Cord Injury in Context

HISTORY

Up to about 40 years ago, the chances of survival of a paraplegic patient were poor, as they had been some 5000 years ago in Egypt, when surgeons first described this condition. Ambrose Pare (1510–1519) was the first modern surgeon to recommend an operation to relieve spinal compression, but it was not until the eighteenth century that the first laminectomy of a fractured spine was performed at St. Thomas's Hospital, London, by the surgeon Henry Cline.

Early in the nineteenth century, Sir Charles Bell, first Dean of the Middlesex Hospital, London, opposed the use of this operation, saying that it was dangerous and useless. He emphasised that all the efforts of a surgeon should be devoted to making an accurate diagnosis initially, maintaining that in cases of paraplegia death was attributable to the retention of the urine and subsequent inflammation of the kidneys. This was the first recorded mention of renal failure being the cause of death. In general, however, there was little advance in the treatment of the condition in the nineteenth century, although progress was made in other directions in the understanding of the condition.

It was World War I that produced a large number of paraplegic patients with gunshot wounds and shrapnel wounds. Although medicine, surgery and nursing had reached a high level of technical skill, and the significance of pressure sores and renal infections was appreciated, the outlook for paraplegics remained grim. It was estimated that the total mortality rate caused by urinary sepsis in British soldiers in World War I was 80%.

Between the two World Wars, despite widespread medical progress in other fields, such as the development of sulphonamides, there were no advances in the treatment of paraplegia, and the prognosis remained hopeless. It was the vision of two men—Donald Munro in the United States in 1936 and Sir Ludwig Guttmann in the United Kingdom in 1944—which transformed the whole outlook for paraplegic patients. They both set up spinal centres where patients were turned regularly so

1

that they did not develop pressure sores, and, by various methods of bladder treatment, they prevented urinary sepsis. They used antibiotics and blood transfusions, keeping the patients alive in the first critical weeks of injury. At a later stage, when the fractured spine had consolidated, they mobilised the patients, teaching them to use the non-paralysed parts of the body, arms and brain to compensate for the paralysed limbs. They taught some patients to walk with calipers, and as a result of their efforts these patients had a nearly normal life-span, participating fully in the life of the community, earning their living in competition with able-bodied people.

Following World War II, specialised centres were set up to deal with patients suffering from traumatic paraplegia. Many of these patients have received specialised care and regular follow-up, so that the natural history of traumatic paraplegia and its complications, as well as methods of rehabilitation and ways of integrating people back into society, have developed considerably in recent years.

The first of these centres in the United Kingdom was set up at Stoke Mandeville Hospital, Aylesbury, Bucks., in 1944 under the direction of Sir Ludwig Guttmann, whose pioneering treatment of people with spinal injuries was so successful that it was designated the National Spinal Injuries Centre in 1951. At this point the centre had 160 beds; it was later expanded to contain 195. Over the years, a number of other units covering the whole of the British Isles opened, and while Stoke Mandeville initially concentrated on war injuries, other units, especially in Sheffield and Wakefield, dealt largely with mining injuries, at least in the early stages.

Over the years, the numbers of people sustaining spinal injuries as the result of war or industrial or mining accidents diminished, but there was no decline in overall prevalence rates, as more people were injured in road traffic and sporting accidents—notably diving and rugby and, more recently, hang-gliding. Accidents in the home involving elderly people are also increasing at present. As the causes of spinal injury have changed over the years, there has also been a change in the incidence of type of injury. The predominance of sporting and motor cycle accidents has resulted in tetraplegia becoming more and paraplegia less common, so that these injuries now occur on an almost equal basis.

There have been a number of changes over the years in the distribution of beds in spinal units throughout England. Stoke Mandeville has reduced in size to 120 beds and moved to a new centre on the same site, the money for which was raised by Jimmy Savile in a national appeal. Two further units have recently opened, at Odstock and Stanmore, leaving the distribution of beds as shown in Table 1.1.

Whether this number and geographical distribution of beds is adequate is an open question. Certainly, a working party of the Royal

Table 1.1　Spinal services

Unit	Available beds	Unit	Available beds
Hexham	30	Pinderfields	30
Lodge Moor	64	Southport	35
Odstock	48	Stanmore	24
Oswestry	46	Stoke Mandeville	120

In addition there are also units in Wales and Scotland.

College of Surgeons accepted the view that there was an adequate number of beds, even if their geographical distribution was less than ideal.

> Although the total number of beds now available for spinal injuries is widely believed to be adequate, and there are no current plans for new units, their size, distribution and staffing are factors so closely related that in relation to future trends and policy they must be considered together. For the development of sufficient expertise amongst the staff, a minimum size must be reached; by contrast, a very large establishment must draw its patients from such a wide area that it becomes remote from the homes of an unacceptable proportion of the patients. Ludwig Guttmann considered that the ideal spinal injuries unit should provide 50 beds; but clearly Stoke Mandeville is very much larger (120) and the most recently opened, Stanmore, currently provides only 24 beds.
>
> (RCS, 1984:5)

However, the South East Thames Regional Health Authority believes that there is sufficient demand for further beds to justify an additional unit in their region. Almost certainly, therefore, there are not enough beds to provide for all the new injuries, and for long-term and follow-up care for those already injured. Further, those people with non-traumatic spinal injuries, who can also gain great benefit from treatment and rehabilitation in a spinal unit, are unlikely to be admitted, given the present number of beds.

TREATMENT AND REHABILITATION

The fundamental principle underlying the rehabilitation of paraplegic patients is to help them help themselves. They do this by using the normal innervated parts of the body to compensate for those parts which are paralysed. To do this effectively, they must be aware of the extent of their injuries at all stages so as to be meaningfully involved in their rehabilitation programmes. The paralysis should not merely be regarded solely as the loss of the normal function of the motor power, the loss of sensation, the loss of bladder and bowel control. The body is more than just a sum of its parts: the paralysed anaesthetic limbs may develop complications such as pressure sores or spasms. These intrude upon a patient's consciousness and well-being and thus impair the function of the whole body.

As a result of the degree of violence usually encountered in a spinal injury, a cord lesion seldom occurs in isolation. It follows that a spinal injury will be associated with injuries to other parts of the body: head injuries in patients with cervical injuries; injury to the thoracic cage and limb fractures in patients with thoracic injuries. Inevitably, such patients are taken from the scene of the accident to a receiving hospital, where they are resuscitated and transferred at a later stage to a spinal centre to complete their rehabilitation. These patients require treatment for at least six months in the early stage and may acquire many of the preventable complications of paraplegia, such as pressure sores and urinary tract infections, if not promptly transferred to a spinal unit.

Once in a spinal unit and with their medical condition stabilised, the rehabilitation process can begin. Patients tend to remain in bed for a few weeks, or sometimes months, until the fracture of the spinal column has stabilised. Then they will be allowed to get up and will be taught to sit and balance properly in their wheelchair. Depending on the level of lesion, patients will be taught to carry out all aspects of self-care, including washing and dressing, management of bladder and bowels, skin care, correct temperature control, and so on. Even where the injury is so severe (high tetraplegics) that these tasks cannot be carried out by the patient concerned, the fundamental principle of rehabilitation remains: that is, the patient is taught to take responsibility for these aspects of his life and to instruct others how to carry them out.

As well as self-care and medical management, there are also broader aspects of the rehabilitation process. The need for a supply of appropriate aids and appliances; the necessity of having adequate means of personal mobility in terms of the right kind of wheelchair and private transport; the issues of housing, employment and income; all need to be addressed. A range of professionals other than doctors will be involved at various stages in this total process, including nurses, physiotherapists, occupational therapists and social workers.

So far we have discussed changes in the medical management of people with spinal injuries, the development of specialist services for people so injured and the principles of their rehabilitation. All of these issues also need to be considered in the context of some of the fundamental changes in ideas and practices which have occurred since World War II in relation to the role and place of disabled people in society.

STATUTORY PROVISION

The framework of statutory provision for disabled people after World War II was laid down by a number of Acts of Parliament, principally the National Health Service Act and the National Assistance Act (1948). These Acts gave local authorities the power to make provision in hospitals or residential units, and to provide aids, equipment and services to meet the needs of disabled people. Further provisions were made in the areas of employment and education by the Education Act (1944) and the Disabled Persons (Employment) Act (1944).

While, in practice, the majority of disabled people have lived and continue to live in the community, from the 1960s onwards two shifts in policy and practice were discernible. First, there was a concern to offer the opportunity for those living in institutions to be reaccommodated within the community, and second, there was a recognition that the quality of life for those disabled people already living in the community needed to be significantly improved. These aims were subsequently encapsulated in a number of legislative changes, most notably the Chronically Sick and Disabled Persons Act (1970), although it is worth pointing out that:

> Had Section 29 of the National Assistance Act been fully implemented and schemes submitted made effective, the history of the disabled would have indeed been different. The seeds of what was later referred to in the House of Commons as 'a charter for the disabled and chronically sick' had already been sown in 1948. Had they fallen on less stony ground the legislation of the seventies might never have been necessary.'
> (Keeble, 1979:35)

In practice, most disabled people were offered the choice between managing in the community, with inadequate support except from their families, and life in an institution or on a hospital ward, which was usually stultifying, restrictive and a threat to dignity and personal identity (Goffman, 1963; Miller and Gwynne, 1971). Such choices were open to people who were spinally injured.

> Depending on domestic circumstances, final discharge may be either to the patient's own home, to institutional care, such as Cheshire Homes or Young Disabled Units, or to a rehabilitation or job re-training centre.
> (Rogers, 1978:85)

Clearly an either/or choice is inadequate to meet the needs of all disabled people, and a number of alternative solutions, such as hostels and half-way houses, have been developed over the years. In the case of those with a spinal injury, for many years the Duchess of Gloucester

House existed as a hostel for paraplegics. It was run by the then Ministry of Labour, and those discharged there were assisted in finding jobs. Other schemes of sheltered accommodation were also developed, including ex-servicemen's homes at the Star and Garter, Richmond, and Chaseley, Sussex, and settlements of bungalows at Lyme Green, Cheshire, and Garston Manor, near Watford. In 1966 a hostel attached to Stoke Mandeville Hospital was opened to offer permanent residence for those tetraplegics who were unable to be discharged elsewhere.

CHANGING IDEAS, CHANGING PRACTICES

However, a number of economic, political and social changes have affected these kinds of provision: notably the economic recession, a political shift to the idea of community care as being the most appropriate form of provision (DHSS, 1968, 1976, 1981) and the struggles of disabled people to assert their rights to live independently.

With regard to the last of these changes, tetraplegics have been in the forefront of the struggle to live independently and have produced accounts of how the problems can be overcome (Davis, 1981; Shearer, 1983; HCIL, 1986). With the acceptance, in theory at least, of the idea that all disabled people have the right to live in the community and with a growing number of successful examples of disabled people successfully so doing, pressure is being put on the statutory authorities from both above and below to provide a more flexible range of services. The old choices between unacceptable institutional care or life within the community, with all the stresses that may place on carers (Briggs and Oliver, 1984), are no longer acceptable.

The question as to whether there is sufficient money, imagination and will to provide the kinds of services needed is beyond the scope of this book, but what we have set out to do is to describe the effects of present service provision on the lives of people with spinal cord injuries and their families. What effect these external changes will have on rehabilitation practices and discharge policies at the spinal units in the United Kingdom remains to be seen, but, as our study will show, there is much that needs to be done.

CHAPTER 2

The Present Study

INTRODUCTION

The purpose of the project described in this book was to carry out an investigation of what has happened to people in the United Kingdom who have experienced a spinal cord injury, for little is known about what has happened to the majority of spinally injured people over the years. Consequently, inadequate attention has been given to the long-term implications of spinal cord injury. It is not known, for example, what impact spinal cord injury has on the processes of personal, family and social life, or what implications it has for employment, or housing, or services. There has been very little published on what happens to people after their injury, what medical problems arise, how life carries on after discharge from hospital and how people cope. The project set out to redress the lack of information currently available about what actually happens to people with spinal cord injury after they leave hospital, to look at this issue in detail, and to explore some of the factors influencing social adjustment. (The full research report has been published separately: Creek *et al.*, 1987.)

There was little prior work on which to build, and so initially we looked for a standarised instrument which would enable us to carry out our research. It was thought that the Social Interview Schedule (SIS) developed at the Institute of Psychiatry would be appropriate for our purposes. Accordingly, some pilot work was carried out, between September 1982 and March 1983. Thirteen people with spinal cord injury were interviewed and the results of this pilot study were written up (Silver *et al.*, 1984). Following on from this work, we decided that the SIS needed to be modified and further instruments developed, to take into account the additional difficulties that may be faced by people with spinal injuries. The main study therefore involved data collection in the following ways: (a) the Social Interview Schedule (modified version); (b) a Spinal Cord Injury Schedule (designed by us); and (c) the General Health Questionnaire (30 point version). These instruments are described more fully elsewhere (Creek *et al.*, 1987). In addition, it was

7

decided to tape-record the interviews, to obtain qualitative as well as quantitative data, as we wanted to study the subjective experience of living with a spinal injury as well as to collect more objective data.

REVIEW OF THE LITERATURE

Little was known, when the study began, about what has happened to the majority of spinally injured people and their families over the years. The National Spinal Injuries Centre (NSIC) has always catered for the after-care of ex-patients, but for various reasons these follow-ups have not been carried out systematically and have not involved all ex-patients. The critical importance of treating newly injured people, lack of resources and the distances that ex-patients may have to travel are all reasons why these follow-ups are not as systematic as they should have been. One study, however, did follow up 125 people discharged from the National Spinal Injuries Centre in 1972, focusing particularly on home care. There were two main conclusions which are of relevance to the present study:

> ... in spite of suitable housing and social services being available to patients returning home after spinal cord injury, only a minority play their optimum role in the community.
>
> The patients seem to divide sharply into two groups. Those who succeed despite enormous difficulties and those who are not able to withstand the pressures of severe disability and often end up disillusioned and resentful.
>
> (Richards, 1975:266)

In the light of the experiences of those we interviewed, both of these conclusions are debatable: housing and social services were not always available, and the division of patients into those who cope and those who do not is an oversimple interpretation of complex issues. However, these issues will be discussed in more detail later.

There have been a number of other studies of various aspects of medical and social life for ex-patients, including a pilot survey by Murray and Thompson (1967) of a Scottish Spinal Injuries Unit. This gave a clear breakdown of the age at which injury occurred, the level of lesion and the cause of injury for those in their region. Regarding their socio-economic status, most of those followed up were working people, although this might possibly differ in regions not centred around one important and hazardous industry. There are a number of inadequacies in the report, however. For instance, many of the measures of 'satisfactory' adjustment in housing or employment were not explicitly defined, and consideration of the views of the individuals and the people around them as to their life-styles was very limited. Nevertheless, the survey raised many interesting issues for further consideration: the possible emotional disadvantages for some people caused by delay in compensation settlement; the importance of 'adequate finance and a feeling of economic security ... to the paraplegic and his immediate circle'; the financial hardship of those dependent on supplementary benefit or old age pension alone; the quality of nursing management in general hospitals; and the problems of ageing relatives and future care. Unfortunately, no attempt to build on this survey had been made until we began our work. Otherwise there has been only a scattering of articles touching on psychosocial issues of spinal cord injury (SCI) in Britain; on sex and marriage (Guttmann, 1964); on sport and the disabled (Guttmann, 1976a); on professional roles and responsibilities in rehabilitation and after-care (Forder *et al.*, 1974); on general practitioner involvement (Mulroy, 1985); and on employment (Goulding, 1976; Marshall and Oliver, 1979).

Far more literature on the psychosocial issues associated with SCI has been published in the United States. The overwhelming focus of attention in this work has been the psychological adjustment of the individual immediately after suffering the injury or shortly after discharge (Siller, 1969; Kerr and Thompson, 1972). Here the predominant model has been one of spinal cord injury as personal tragedy, where the individual sufferer is expected to pass through a series of stages of adjustment closely akin to the processes involved in bereavement: grief or mourning, shock, denial, anger and depression. Any questioning or rebellion against the aims and methods of rehabilitation proffered or failure to reach the rehabilitation goals is usually, therefore, interpreted as an individual failure in adjustment, and account is rarely taken of the family context of adjustment to the injury or the wider social situation.

These works have been scrutinised by Trieschmann (1980), who concludes that little evidence has been produced to substantiate this model. She finds no evidence to show that these stages of psychological adjustment do occur, whereas studies have shown that rehabilitation staff, who have frequently been called upon to make such assessments, consistently overestimate the degree of psychological stress felt by patients. In addition, as those experiencing SCI are not a homogeneous group, individual reactions are likely to differ, depending on a number of other factors, such as family background, socio-economic group, age, and so on.

Furthermore, Trieschmann (1980) points out that most of the research has focused on the characteristics of the individual, identifying those who adapt successfully but without addressing the problem of how to help the large number of apparent failures. She severely criticises the use in a number of studies of a criterion of attainment of full-time employment as a measure of success, arguing that this is only one of many behaviours in life. The very terms 'adjustment', 'success' and 'rehabilitation' are shown to be difficult to interpret, with no agreement to date on their meanings. To avoid such errors in judgement and interpretation, she proposes that data must be amassed on what people actually do following rehabilitation, in order to have a basis for comparison and to begin to evaluate the effect of rehabilitative treatment. Trieschmann also highlights considerable evidence that the behaviour of disabled people is greatly influenced by their environment, by their individual, social and physical situations, and by wider aspects of policy and provision, including factors such as the range of services available and the expectations of others about an appropriate role for disabled people in society.

A recent study looking at long-term adjustment found that:

> ... persons who have high levels of social support, who are satisfied with their social contacts and who feel they have high levels of perceived control report high levels of well-being.
>
> (Schulz and Decker, 1985:1162)

A further study of 166 people with spinal cord injury in Australia came up with a list of priorities as reported by the people with spinal cord injury themselves (Table 2.1). Similarly, an evaluation of one year's referrals to the Welfare Service of the Spinal Injuries Association in Great Britain (Hasler and Oliver, 1982) showed that the major concerns were related to the physical and social environments rather than to individual medical or psychological problems.

Table 2.1 List of priorities: self-reported (%)

Accommodation	59	Financial and legal	9
Employment	15	Sexuality	5
Transport	14	Leisure	4
Equipment and assistance	19	Sport	3

Adapted from Richards, 1982:91.

Clearly, then, conceptual frameworks provided by the 'psychological model theorists', which stress the need for psychological adjustment as a progression through a series of stages (Weller and Miller, 1977) which the individual must pass, have a number of inadequacies. One of us has provided a number of criticisms of this approach.

Firstly, the model of man which these theories implicitly draws upon is one where man is determined by the things that happen to him—the adjustment to disability can only be achieved by experiencing a number of these psychological mechanisms or by working through a number of fixed stages. Secondly, adjustment is seen as largely an individual phenomenon, a problem for the disabled person, and as a consequence, the family context and the wider social situation are neglected. Finally, such explanations fail to accord with the personal reality of many disabled people, particularly those with traumatic spinal cord injury, who may not grieve or mourn or pass through a series of adjustment stages.

(Oliver, 1981:50)

Finkelstein goes further than criticism of psychological models. He argues that disability is a social relationship and he insists that:

... disability is viewed as a paradoxical situation involving the state of the individual (his or her impairment) and the state of society (the social restrictions which are imposed on the individual)...

(Finkelstein, 1980:6)

An individual's material circumstances are crucial to how his or her disability will be experienced. However, the relationship between the individual and society cannot simply be understood as a function of the degree of impairment of an individual and the extent of the social restriction that impaired individuals face. There is an intervening variable which needs to be considered, which can be called 'meaning':

The experiences which individuals have, the things that happen to them, are not fixed or stable, but rather take the form of a process through which individuals can negotiate their own passages. Further, these negotiated passages are not determined by events that occur (like paralysis as the result of an accident) but only by the meanings that individuals attach to these occurrences. These meanings are not themselves solely the product of individual consciousness, but arrived at as the result of interactions with other people, close relatives and friends and the public at large.

(Oliver, 1981:52)

CONCEPTUAL FRAMEWORK

For us, then, understanding the consequences of SCI involves a complex relationship between the impaired individual, the social context within which the impairment occurs and the meanings available to individuals to enable them to make sense of what is happening. This is what we mean by social adjustment: it is more than simply the functional limitations that an individual has or the social restrictions encountered;

it is a complex relationship between impairment, social restrictions and meaning.

In attempting to provide an adequate conceptual framework, we were not convinced about the dominant view of spinal cord injury as a personal tragedy. Clearly, breaking one's back or neck may have tragic consequences for some individuals, but, as most people appear to cope with such a happening, such coping, therefore, can only be explained by reference to such unscientific (and unhelpful) notions as the indomitable nature of the human spirit. This gives rise to the 'supercripple' phenomenon in which those who cope are ascribed with heroic characteristics. This flies in the face of the everyday realities of people with spinal cord injury, who see themselves as ordinary people coping with extraordinary circumstances.

Another view, recently articulated by a number of disabled people themselves (UPIAS, 1976), sees disability as nothing more than social oppression—the social restrictions imposed upon impaired individuals by an uncaring or unknowing society. Again, clearly, this view is inadequate, for having a spinal cord injury imposes a number of personal problems, such as bladder and bowel incontinence, urinary infections, risk of pressure sores, and so on, which cannot be explained in terms of social oppression.

Within the field of medical sociology, there is a great deal of literature and published research which uses 'life events' as a conceptual framework. Much of this work has focused on distressing or negative life events (Mechanic, 1962), although it has been argued (Dohrenwend and Dohrenwend, 1974) that there is no need for life events to be seen in this way. For Dohrenwend and Dohrenwend, the important characteristic of a life event is that it should be disrupting or have the potential to disrupt. Thus, a wide range of life events can be studied, including leaving school, starting a job, getting married, having a child, obtaining a divorce, being made redundant and dying. What makes life events significant is the meanings attached to them, for:

> It is likely to be the meaning of events that is significant rather than change as such.
>
> (Brown and Harris, 1979:66)

A massive review of the American literature on coping with significant life events, in which spinal cord injury is included, suggests:

> Our review of the available literature suggests that a great deal of variability exists in individual reactions to negative life events, both within a particular life crisis and across different crises. We have found little reliable evidence to indicate that people go through stages of emotional responses following an undesirable life event. We have also

reviewed a substantial body of evidence suggesting that a large minority of victims of aversive life events experience distress or disorganization long after recovery might be expected. Current theoretical models of reactions to aversive outcomes cannot account for the variety of responses that appear.

(Silver and Wortman, 1980:309)

That spinal cord injury constitutes a significant life event there can be no doubt and the above quotation provides a reasonable introduction to and summary of our own data, to be presented subsequently. Existing models, whether they be individual (personal tragedy theory) or social (social oppression theory) cannot cope with the range and variety of our data, and the concept of significant life event appears to be the only one available to take account of individual impairment, social context and meaning.

We also utilised the concept of career because we wished to consider spinal cord injury over time and not just as a one-off event. In addition, the meaning of SCI was an intervening variable between the extent of the individual's physical impairment and his or her social and material circumstances. Career combines these two things, for, as one researcher has noted of her own study:

. . . the 'career' perspective for this study offered two advantages. Firstly, it enabled some account to be taken of the dimension of time and, secondly, it facilitated movement between the 'micro' and the 'macro', the structure and the action.

(Blaxter, 1980:248)

Before proceeding to consider our own data within this conceptual framework, it is necessary that we provide a brief description of some of the characteristics of the people we interviewed.

CHARACTERISTICS OF THE PEOPLE INTERVIEWED

A sampling frame consisting of 550 people admitted by one consultant to one of the acute wards of the National Spinal Injuries Centre was used. These people were admitted between the years 1971 and 1984, and a one-in-four sample was extracted on a chronological basis. Because, initially, this consultant only treated males, females were not included in the sampling frame, although a similar study of women with spinal cord injury is clearly needed. It was felt that by using ex-patients from one consultant, differential treatment patterns would not influence the data. Details of those selected from the sampling frame were taken from medical records retained by the Spinal Injuries Unit. These records were not always complete or up to date, and often did not contain most recent addresses or correct information about a person's doctor. Consequently, compilation of demographic information took a great deal of time and ingenuity. The Family Practitioner Committees provided information on the whereabouts of several people. Once the necessary details had been obtained, contact was made with the GP and as many as possible of the ex-patients were contacted by letter and asked whether they would like to take part in an interview. Table 2.2 shows the proportion of those who agreed to be interviewed, and also the reasons for non-participation.

Table 2.2   Participation/non-participation pattern for total sample

Category	Number	Percentage
Agreed to interview	77	56
No trace	19	13.8
Dead	20	14.8
Distance prohibitive	4	2.9
Not contacted	1	1
Refusal—too ill	4	2.9
Refusal—other reason known	7	5.1
Refusal—reason unknown	5	3.6
	137	100

Of 137 selected for interview, we were unable to trace 19 despite following up through the Family Practitioner Clinic, the Post Office and sometimes relatives or neighbours. Thus, we have no idea of what the long-term effects of spinal cord injury might have been for 14% of our sample population. A further 20 whom we did trace were found to have died, and a further person was reported by an ex-neighbour to have died, although this was unconfirmed. Two people had moved out of the country and thus could not be interviewed, and one other person lived too far away for us to meet. One person whom it was not possible to arrange to meet sent a tape-recording of his experiences based around the interview schedule. One person was in hospital at the time of contact and we decided that it would be inappropriate to suggest an interview. Sixteen people refused to take part in the research. Of these, four refused because they were too ill—two were actually in hospital at the time, and one was awaiting his twenty-seventh operation since being injured. Five people said that they did not feel up to taking part at the time, and a further five did not want to be interviewed, for unknown reasons. One person was too busy to take part because he was in the process of moving house. Ultimately, 77 people—65% of those alive at the time of contact—agreed to be interviewed: that is, 56% of the total sample.

It is striking that 20 people from our original sample had died and that a further 19 could not be traced. Thus, a mortality rate of at least 14% (the number of deaths among those untraced is unknown) has medical implications worthy of further investigation. It may also have legal implications regarding claims for compensation, in that the risk of death from spinal cord injury is perhaps higher than had previously been supposed. A similar percentage of people who have disappeared is clearly worrying for those concerned to provide after-care and follow-up for those with a spinal injury.

The length of time since people had received their injuries ranged from 10 months to 14 years. About a third had received their injury in the 4 years prior to interview; another third, between 5 and 9 years earlier; and a third, 10 or more years ago. Age at injury ranged from 15 to 67 years. Approximately a third were aged 20 or less and slightly more than half were under 23 at the time of injury. Only 5% of those interviewed were aged 60 or more when they were injured. At the time of being interviewed, their ages ranged between 20 and 77 years and just over half were in their early thirties or younger. A fuller breakdown is given in Tables 2.3–2.5.

We interviewed slightly more paraplegics (with thoracic, lumbar or sacral lesions—53%) than tetraplegics (with cervical lesions—47%).

Table 2.3   Age at injury

Age	Number	Percentage
0–19	21	27.3
20–24	19	24.7
25–34	14	18.2
35–44	8	10.4
45–54	10	13.0
55+	5	6.5
	77	100

Table 2.4   Current age

Age	Number	Percentage
0–24	14	18.2
25–34	28	36.4
35–44	17	22.1
45–59	9	11.7
60+	9	11.7
	77	100

Table 2.5 Length of time since injury

Years	Number	Percentage
0–4	23	29.9
5–9	28	36.4
10–15	26	33.8
	77	100

Table 2.6 Types of lesion of respondents ($N = 77$)

Degree of completeness	Level	Percentage
Complete	Tetraplegic	18
Incomplete	Tetraplegic	28
Complete	Paraplegic	31
Incomplete	Paraplegic	18
Incomplete/complete	Higher/lower	5

Almost half of the lesions were complete (40%), just under half were incomplete (46%), and the remaining few were incomplete at a higher level and complete at lower level. Table 2.6 summarises the degree of completeness and level of lesion of the 77 people interviewed.

Causes of spinal injury were varied. Table 2.7 gives a breakdown of the cause of injury for our sample. Half of the people interviewed had received their injury as a result of road traffic accidents, mainly involving cars or motorcycles, and one person had been injured as a pedestrian. Most of those involved in traffic accidents were driving at the time. Table 2.8 gives a breakdown of the different types of road traffic accidents in which injuries were sustained. Amateur sporting accidents comprised the next major cause of injury, and there was one professional sporting injury. Rugby, hang-gliding and diving were the sporting activities most frequently associated with injury. A further group had received industrial injuries or had been injured at work. There was some overlap here with injuries sustained in traffic accidents where vehicles were involved—for example, lorry-driving accidents. Accidents in the home accounted for a small percentage of spinal injuries, and there was one self-inflicted injury. Finally, there was a small group of people whose injuries were caused by falls that neither involved vehicles nor occurred in the home. Clearly, spinal injuries of medical origin are underrepresented in our sample, and this may well have resulted from a combination of the acute ward chosen and the manner of referrals and admissions of those people with non-traumatic spinal cord lesions.

Table 2.7 Causes (%) of spinal injury for total sample (*N* = 77)

Road traffic accident	50
Amateur sporting injury	23
Professional sporting injury	1
Industrial/work injury	10
Accidents in the home	8
Falls	3
Self-inflicted injury	1
Medical onset	4

Table 2.8 Types of road traffic acidents involving injury

Nature of Accident	Percentage	Victim's status	Percentage
Car	50	Driver	78
Motor cycle	42	Passenger	22
Lorry/van	5	*N* = 5	
Pedestrian	3		
N = 38			

At the time of interview exactly half of the sample were single, and 38% were either married or cohabiting. A small number were divorced or separated (10%). One person was widowed. A rough breakdown of the geographical location of the people we interviewed showed that most lived in towns (41%) or cities, including London (33%). A fairly large group lived in villages or rural areas (26%).

Interviews were carried out usually, but not necessarily, in people's own homes. This was thought to be more conducive to a full and frank interview than interviewing in the hospital setting. In the specific conditions of this investigation, where mobility and distance from the Spinal Injuries Unit were critical factors, interviewing in the home also enabled people from a wider population to be contacted. In addition, a relative or friend was invited to be present if the interviewee wished. In such situations a joint interview was conducted in which the person with a spinal injury was the main focus of attention. The role of the other person was to substantiate information given about objective circumstances, and to supplement the responses concerning management and satisfaction.

Forty-seven of the interviews were with the person on his own (61%). Where someone else was also present, in nine cases it was the wife of the spinally injured person (22%) and in seven cases the parent (9%). On a few occasions another member of the family or another person, not necessarily related, took part. In those interviews where others were present, they were not necessarily there all the time but may have called in or out at different times. The interviews lasted on average 3 hours, although those with newly discharged ex-patients were sometimes shorter, being completed in 1½ hours.

CONCLUSIONS

This chapter, then, has provided a description of the research project, reviewed the relevant literature on spinal cord injury, laid down a conceptual framework in which to locate our data, and briefly described some of the characteristics of those we interviewed. What follows will develop the idea of a career in spinal cord injury and will utilise the concepts of social adjustment and significant life events.

CHAPTER 3

The Medical Consequences
of Spinal Injury

INTRODUCTION

Medical aspects of the disability career with regard to spinal injury follow three stages.

First, the person concerned will have damaged his spinal cord in an accident and will then usually be admitted to the nearest receiving hospital, where he will be initially assessed and treated.

Second, he will be transferred from the receiving hospital to a specialist spinal unit, sometimes within a few hours or days, although on other occasions it may take weeks or even months. The time taken to transfer depends on a number of factors: the treatment of life-threatening complications (particularly respiratory failure), other medical complications, the availability of beds, the inclination of the consultant concerned. Early transfer to a spinal unit is the best policy for all concerned, for district hospitals are inexperienced in dealing with spinal injury in combination with severe associated injuries. It is vital not only that complications be prevented, but also that a positive approach be made to the patient and his family about the likely outcome with regard to work, housing and the difficult psychosocial adjustments.

> Since the war, when the great majority of traumatic cord injuries have been due to closed fractures or fracture-dislocations, patients have been admitted in ever-increasing numbers either immediately or within the first few days after injury from casualty departments of general hospitals, or from accident, neurosurgical or orthopaedic hospitals. This has been more and more recognised by surgeons as the most satisfactory procedure to avoid early infection of the paralysed bladder and the development of other complications, especially pressure sores . . . .
>
> (Guttmann, 1976b)

Once in the spinal unit and with the medical condition stabilised, attention is then directed to the care of the skin, the bladder and the bowels, and the prevention of complications such as pressure sores, urinary infections and muscle contractures. Patients will be turned regularly, intermittent catheterisation and bladder wash-outs may take place, and regular physiotherapy will be provided while the patient is still in bed. The rehabilitation process will start while the patient is still in bed, with occupational therapy and physiotherapy, and after a period varying between a few weeks and several months, he will be got up into a wheelchair and rehabilitation will begin in earnest.

After this process is complete, the third stage in the disability career will be reached and the person concerned will be discharged back to the community. It is hoped that the rehabilitation process will have taught the person how to look after the skin, bladder, bowels and paralysed muscles and to recognise any medical complications that may arise from time to time.

Unfortunately, however, the necessary skills and knowledge may not exist within the local health authority, for, as has been pointed out:

> The long-term management of paraplegics and tetraplegics in their own home thus demands a wider dissemination of the skills required for spinal injury than is at present available.
>
> (RCS, 1984:6)

Thus, the spinal units provide a regular check-up and after-care service to ex-patients, but not everyone takes advantage of this or is able to gain readmission when necessary.

This three-stage disability career will provide the framework into which our material is organised in this chapter. First, therefore, we will consider the experiences people had in the receiving hospital, immediately after the accident.

EXPERIENCES AT RECEIVING HOSPITALS

A considerable range of experiences were reported to us, and while some people received a great deal of skilled attention and support, the majority reported that the level of specialist knowledge of spinal injury and how to treat it was low. In some cases this lack of adequate knowledge had serious medical consequences, such as aggravation of the injury through inappropriate handling, the development of pressure sores and damage to the kidneys.

These reports of experiences prior to transfer raise a number of important issues. For some, failure to receive specialist treatment at the receiving hospital gave rise to medical and physical problems that persisted over long periods of time. One man who spent 6 weeks in a general hospital before transfer could be arranged explained that during this time:

My limbs started to go tight, I got frozen shoulders and I paid the price for the next two years.

Lack of specialist knowledge, sometimes coupled with insensitivity on the part of professionals, often gave rise to medical complications for those experiencing transfer delay, as the following comments convey:

> I told them I'd broken my back and they took no notice. They seemed to think they knew better. They sat me up and pulled my jumper off over my head. I asked them then to cut it off—they took no notice—they said: 'how do you know you've broken your back?'—That's what annoyed me more than anything. Then they X-rayed me and told me I'd broken my back. After four days I had bed sores—they'd put me on a solid board and didn't turn me. I had blisters on my heels ... I often wonder if I'd be better off now if they'd handled me better. I had a bad transfer. I was almost dead when I got to Stoke. I was blue and my stomach wasn't working.

Another man reported 'a terrible three weeks trying to walk in a Zimmer frame', not knowing he had broken his back.

Failure to diagnose the spinal cord injury frequently characterised non-specialist initial provision. One person, again in a general hospital, explained:

> They didn't diagnose the broken neck until it started to swell, and I complained of pain when I came to, and then they started to treat it. But during that time it had swollen up so bad that it was cutting off everything and affecting my breathing.

Those for whom the first place of admission was not in the United Kingdom could experience particular problems. A man injured in Argentina recalled being told in hospital to walk home, and that he would probably wake up with a sore neck—he was subsequently paralysed on waking. This man had then been admitted to a British hospital, still in Argentina, where he developed 'massive pressure sores', resulting in an eventual 2½ year stay at the NSIC. Similarly, a young man serving in the RAF in America described how in retrospect he realised that at his initial hospital 'the people didn't have a clue what they were doing'. He was, erroneously, told that he would walk within a year of injury, and this initial mistaken prognosis was said to have fostered psychological and emotional difficulties for several years after. In addition, both described transfer flights to the United Kingdom as uncomfortable, claustrophobic and extremely distressing.

TRANSFER TO THE SPINAL UNIT

Table 3.1 shows that over half of those interviewed were transferred to the spinal unit at Stoke Mandeville Hospital within 2 weeks of their

Table 3.1 Length of time taken to transfer to spinal
unit after injury

Time	Number	Percentage
Same day	3	4
1–2 days	12	16
3–7 days	15	20
1–2 weeks	12	16
2–3 weeks	6	8
3–4 weeks	5	6
4–6 weeks	5	6
6–8 weeks	6	8
Longer	12	16
	76	100

Missing cases = 1.

injury. Over 75% were transferred within 6 weeks. The total period of
hospitalisation ranged from 6 months to over a year for a small number
of people. Nearly 70% were discharged within 8 months, with between
4 and 8 months being the most common length of stay.

One particularly interesting feature of the responses during the
interviews was that people's experiences in the receiving hospital often
significantly influenced their anticipatory perception of the spinal unit
and what was awaiting them when they got there. One particularly
unfortunate consequence of this situation is that some respondents were
led to believe that their injuries were not as serious as they in fact were.
As we have already suggested, to have a spinal cord injury is a
significant life event, but *when* this life event actually becomes significant
is a crucial question. People struggle to understand the meaning of what
has happened to them and have to cope with the uncertainty of not
knowing the precise details. The following quotations from three
different individuals indicate some of the dimensions of this struggle for
meaning.

They really did not know or if they did know they were reluctant to tell
me the actual truth of the matter. They effectively led me to believe that I
would be at Stoke for four or five weeks, then would be back home
without any problems, so it was a bit of a blow when I got to Stoke and
found out that wasn't quite how things would work out.

Nobody ever told me about bowels and things like that; they didn't tell
you about the bladder. They didn't give you any information at all—it
wasn't until I went to Stoke Mandeville that I found out about all these
things.

Nobody had told me I was going to be a cripple for the rest of my life or
anything of that nature. Actually, in the first instance I thought I was

going to get well again; they were trying to make me walk—they didn't tell me what was the matter with me until I went to Stoke Mandeville.

The reluctance or hesitation to inform people about the extent of their injuries contrasts quite markedly with the way in which this situation was handled at the spinal unit: the adding of significance to the life event, so to speak. Practically all recalled that their consultant's prognosis was very direct and, usually, given within one or two days of arrival. However, this direct approach produced very mixed reactions among some individuals. In some cases, as the extracts above suggest, finding out about the extent of their injuries produced a feeling of shock. This was often accompanied by a certain resentment and the feeling that the issue should be handled with more sensitivity.

> I was wheeled into the [consultant's] room and treated really as though, I don't know, something awful, something that was not even a human being.
>
>   Poking and prodding and then basically told—'tough luck, buster—you'll not be walking again with your legs but we may be able to do something for you with some other implements'—well, it was rather, to say the least, a disturbing way I was treated. I'll never forget that as long as I live . . . well, fair enough, the facts were there and I can understand that, and obviously that comes hard to anybody but it was just the way you are treated as just a piece of meat if you like. It was horrible, a horrible experience.

In retrospect, however, even those who experienced initial resentment often subsequently expressed appreciation that at least they had not been misled by false optimism.

> I think it's a good idea that you were told—the rest of your life is involved, so the quicker you get resigned to it the better.

> I only understood about the injury very gradually—I was very woozy at the time. I remember talking to him [the consultant] and he was very adamant it was a complete and permanent injury and that there was no hope of any recovery or anything—I think that upset me at the time, but when I look back on it now, I can understand why he did it and I think it was the right thing to do.

These extracts from the interview data suggest that, while there may be no single 'right way' to inform people about the extent of their injury, an early prognosis is generally preferable to the hesitation or misinformation experienced in some of the receiving hospitals. Many people who reported such experiences also recalled a feeling of relief when the situation was confirmed. This is well illustrated by one person who reported only being told 'bits and pieces' in the receiving hospital:

> I think I knew or suspected most of it. He [the consultant] just said—'Do you understand what's happened to you?'—He didn't make a fuss about it or anything, he just confirmed my doubts.... On the whole it was handled well, people didn't keep you guessing or tell you half-truths to help your feelings, but I don't remember it too well.

In our terms, the meaning of the life event had been made significant. But, of course, there is more to being in the spinal unit at Stoke Mandeville Hospital than how someone is told of his injury. There is general agreement that specialist spinal units are very good at providing people with the information necessary to take care of skin, bladder, bowels and paralysed muscles, so we do not propose to provide data on this aspect. It is also usually assumed that the rehabilitation process is excellent, but a number of people we interviewed did not fully endorse this view. A major criticism centred around the inflexibility of the regime, as the following quotations illustrate.

> Their attitude is so regimental—you've got to do this, 'If you don't like our treatment, goodbye'.

> At Stoke there is an inertia—[the attitude is] we have developed this system of rehabilitation as if it were engraved in tablets of stone—the system is so inflexible—the patients just slot in.

Others found the rehabilitation to be a great practical benefit.

> In Stoke they gave you the golden rule—the golden method—that was it, you went out and followed that for the rest of your life. You can tell someone who has been rehabilitated at Stoke a mile away by the way they did things.

There were also criticisms of omission, in that there was a failure to meet people's emotional and psychological needs:

> It was all on a practical level. There was virtually nothing on a mental level.

> The time spent on the psychological side was minimal.

These criticisms were criticisms of the regime itself rather than of individual staff members.

> Despite my criticisms of Stoke, there were a lot of nice people who *cared*. When you are lying in bed for a long time it's very easy to become an inmate—I know a lot of people who dreaded leaving.... I felt a lot of people treated you like an individual, but the system didn't—OK, you accept there have got to be procedures but within that, the little personal touch wasn't always there.

Obviously, a degree of regimentation is almost inevitable in any large organisation such as a hospital. However, these extracts illustrate that while there is no lack of skilled care within the spinal unit, many respondents perceived such care as particularly 'de-personalising'. Although individual members of staff at the spinal units were often highly supportive, this did not necessarily mitigate the overall regimentation with which services within the unit were delivered.

Despite the various problems associated with the services at the spinal unit, most people appreciated that the specialist care they had received there was superior to that provided by other hospitals:

> At the time at Stoke Mandeville Hospital, one thought that what was said and what was done for you wasn't necessary—they were being sort of hard on you and all that . . . it's only after you leave that you realise what they have said, what they have done for you has been the best medical attention in the world—what they have done, the facilities, the rehabilitation, the advice and the doctors—it's the best . . . you only realise that afterwards.

As this extract illustrates, such perceptions of the unit often emerged retrospectively—particularly if ex-patients had had unsatisfactory experiences when readmitted to other hospitals for check-ups or other treatment. A quantitative indication of the trend is given in Table 3.2. Table 3.3 shows that people's preference for the spinal unit over other hospitals was even more marked in relation to general rehabilitation.

Table 3.2   Choice of hospital for readmission

Hospital	Number	Percentage
SIU	46	63.0
Other	9	12.3
SIU if spinal cord-related	12	16.4
Don't know	6	8.3
	73	100

Missing cases = 4.

Table 3.3   Preference for rehabilitation

Hospital	Number	Percentage
SIU	54	76.1
Other	5	7.0
Don't know	12	16.9
	71	100

Missing cases = 6.

DISCHARGE INTO THE COMMUNITY

The third stage in this part of the disability career occurs when it is time to be discharged from the spinal unit. The majority of patients usually return to their own homes or to some form of statutory provision, and issues arising in this area will be discussed in more detail in Chapter 7. However, it is not always possible for adaptations or statutory provision to be organised on a suitable basis at the time of discharge and it has been estimated that as many as 20% of spinal beds may be blocked at any one time because there is no suitable place for discharge (RCS, 1984).

For some this may mean discharge to a non-specialist hospital nearer their place of residence. Medical and physical difficulties, reminiscent of those related to non-specialist initial or intermediate treatment, sometimes arose. The following comments relate to 6 months spent in a general hospital immediately after discharge from the spinal unit, necessitated by the failure of a local council to provide adequate housing.

> They just weren't equipped to deal with me. They didn't know anything about me. I had a very bad time and got to the point that I just didn't want to live any more. Well I did want to live . . . I never gave up exactly, but that was where I realised that if this was how it was going to be I'm not sure I want to go on. They didn't know how to do my bowels or bladder and I was having three or four accidents a week as far as bowels and bladder were concerned, and it was just getting too much, all of it. I thought that was the way it was going to be, and that was how tetraplegics lived until I found out it wasn't the way it had to be at all . . .
>
> Just before I left, at the end of 14 months, I developed a very small sore which unfortunately they never told me about. I was leaving 2 days afterwards and I think they knew it was there but they didn't want to tell me because they knew I was going home, but it put me in bed for the first 5 weeks of being home, which made it even worse.

It is clear, therefore, that serious problems can arise as a result of non-specialised medical provision after discharge as well as before admission to a spinal unit.

Medical problems or complications which necessitate readmission to the spinal unit may also arise for those discharged to their own homes or statutory provision. Almost 60% of the sample reported at least one readmission. Table 3.4 gives the number of reported readmissions of those stating they had readmissions, including those for respite care. It can be seen that 67% of those reporting readmissions had been readmitted on two or more occasions.

Pressure sores and bladder infections comprise the two major reasons for readmissions. Other reasons for readmission were varied, and include further rehabilitation, spinal cysts, broken legs, tendon

Table 3.4 Number of reported readmissions[a] of those stating they had readmissions

Readmissions	Number	Percentage
1	15	32.6
2	12	26.1
3	7	15.2
4	5	10.9
6	2	4.3
7	1	2.2
Repeated number (not specified)	4	8.7
	46	100

[a]Includes respite care.

transplants, and so on. Given the high percentage of people reporting readmissions to hospital, it is useful to consider some of the comments made about this during the interviews.

Several people reported readmissions to hospital within a relatively short period of initial discharge. A few people reported a series of repeated readmissions during this time, indicative of medical complications in the early years, which were more serious for some than for others. One man, for example, gave the following reasons for a series of subsequent readmissions within 2 years of injury: first, to have screws, put in place at the time of injury, removed from his neck; second, because of thrombosis; and third, because of bladder problems and to have a bladder implant. Another person described how medical complications had arisen only months after discharge and had continued up to the present time, 4 years after injury:

> About 9 months after being discharged I got a small infection in my groin on the inside of my leg. It got a little bit worse, and basically, probably through my own fault initially, I was eventually admitted under the surgeons at [a major London teaching hospital] when I was quite ill, about a month after this had started. I was in [the teaching hospital] 8 months as a patient, gradually deteriorating. I had several operations to try and clear this thing up. Eventually they did an operation on my hip joint because it was infected. Eventually, Dr Silver came at the request of one of the registrars at the teaching hospital—or maybe a consultant—and he came and saw me and took me [back] into Stoke Mandeville. I had my hip joint removed by the orthopaedic surgeon there but that didn't clear up the infection entirely and I still had a discharge and so on after that. I went back to see the orthopaedic surgeon again on several occasions. He said that there wasn't much more he could do.

This person's GP arranged for him to be admitted to a second spinal injuries unit, but medical complications persisted:

I wasn't admitted to the spinal unit because I was infected, but to the Infectious Diseases Unit, where they did a further operation on the hip to remove the rest of the dead bone and infected tissue. I was there another 3½ months. I'll just go through it: September 1981—discharged; Summer 1982—back in hospital; March 1983—out again; April 1984—back in again and to another spinal unit; October 1984—out again; and I've been out ever since. Nearly a year. This is my first year out. I've been in more than out.

While this is the most dramatic example of problems occurring shortly after discharge from the spinal unit, a few people reported continuing ill-health for at least 2 years after discharge and four people who refused to take part in the study did so because of ill-health. Others reported skin breakdown and bladder infections in the immediate post-discharge period, and one person reported that:

I really haven't been well enough to do anything, hobbies, etc ... I've really only been taking one day at a time.

Not all medical complications necessitated readmission to hospital, but some meant that individuals were confined to bed in their own homes. Tables 3.5 and 3.6 give the numbers of those reporting

Table 3.5   Number of times confined to bed at home

Times	Number	Percentage
1 occasion	17	46.0
2 occasions	8	21.6
3 occasions	5	13.5
5 occasions	2	5.4
8 or more/repeated	5	13.5
	37	100

Missing cases = 3.

Table 3.6   Reported reasons for first confinement to bed at home

Reason	Number	Percentage
Pressure sore	17	43
Bladder infection	5	13
Kidney infection	1	2
Marks on skin	5	12
Other	8	20
Combinations	4	10
	40	100

confinements to bed at home for conditions relating to spinal injury, since initial discharge from hospital, and illustrate the reported reasons for confinement. Again, it will be noted from Table 3.6 that the major causes of confinement to bed were the same as for hospital readmissions—pressure sores and bladder problems, including infections—and this pattern was similar for second, third and subsequent confinements to bed.

People were asked whether they had regular physical check-ups and half said that they did have regular physical check-ups, whereas almost the same number said that they did not. As a general rule, everyone receives an initial check-up 6 weeks after discharge. Until recently, however, NSIC has only responded to requests for check-ups rather than institute a regular system of follow-ups for all. Many people wanted a more regular system of follow-up, but for some the travelling distances involved acted as a barrier to regular self-referral for check-ups. A small group of those interviewed had not been discharged for a long enough period of time to have established a pattern of check-ups. Table 3.7 illustrates these findings. Table 3.8 indicates the locations of regular physical check-ups for those who said that they had them: 50% took place at the National Spinal Injuries Unit. A small proportion of check-ups were at other spinal units, with slightly fewer at other hospitals or with GPs.

Table 3.7   Regular physical check-ups

Category	Number	Percentage
Yes	38	50
No	33	43.4
Not applicable (too soon)	5	6.6
	76	100

Missing cases = 1.

Table 3.8   Location of physical check-ups

Location	Number	Percentage
NSIU	19	50.0
Different SIU	5	13.2
SIU and other	4	10.5
Local hospital	1	2.6
GP	5	13.2
Other	4	10.5
	38	100

We asked not just about medical problems that may have arisen after discharge, but also about further aspects of the rehabilitation and recovery process. People were asked briefly what they were able to do physically on discharge from hospital in terms of mobility, bladder and bowel management, and personal care. They were also asked about their present physical abilities, if there had been any change from those on discharge. Obviously, there could have been a problem for some people of exact recall of their physical capabilities at the time they left hospital. However, many did note that although they had little change in their physical recovery over the years, they had become stronger with time. For instance, one stated:

> I've had absolutely no recovery since I left Stoke Mandeville but what I have been left with has got stronger.

Those who reported little change in their abilities were often people with complete lesions. Some people with incomplete lesions recorded certain improvements in their physical abilities over the first year or two. In one or two cases the people themselves noted that it was only after this period of sometimes intensive physiotherapy or exercise that they themselves came to the realisation that they had probably achieved as much improvement in their physical abilities as they felt, by then, likely to achieve. One person said:

> During the 2 years after I went home I had been told that I would probably go on improving but after 2 years your condition stabilised so I went bananas really. I went back to work and everything but I was going to physio two or three times a week, mostly for hydrotherapy at our local hospital. I was doing exercises at home—a couple of hours a day, I was going like mad at that because I thought—right, if I've got a couple of years I'll try and get normal, because I was very hopeful really of making a full recovery. As time went by you saw the months slipping away and the 2 years approaching. I wasn't actually improving that much . . . you know I wasn't normal. And then the old depression started to seep in and at that stage the GP was very helpful because he said: 'Look, you are going to have to accept how you are. You know you've been trying very hard and you've done very well but you need to accept how you are.' And that was a pretty large moment of truth really and it began to dawn on me that I was not going to be normal and I think I had been hoping for that. I think he could see what was happening and he understood me and was very helpful.

Another reported that there had been actual improvement in his toe movement but noted that although this gave him hope, it was not of any actual functional benefit. One person, however, did describe some quite significant changes in his ability to move muscles and feel sensation as much as 5 years after his injury. He noted that this was predominantly on his right side and although it had brought some functional return, he also stressed that it was causing him some discomfort. In particular, he complained that the root pain which had always previously been constant had become more powerful since the regeneration. The issue of pain was one that was recurrent in many interviews, and will be discussed a little later.

For a number of people, coping with double incontinence was a major difficulty. Indeed, one or two people, most notably those older respondents at the time of injury, cited this as their major concern. Problems with urinal incontinence were compounded by the problems a number of people had had over many years with bladder infections. One person noted that he had had repeated bladder infections over the years, although he no longer stayed in bed for them:

> It's a minor detail now—you just don't bother about it—you just feel absolutely rotten for a week—I don't take antibiotics because they don't agree with me.

Usually, difficulties concerning the bladder and urinary incontinence seemed to be surmountable over time and with certain treatments. For some, the problems of coping with bowel management were longer-lasting and far more of a concern. Some people noted the distress, frustration or simply annoyance caused by the amount of time it took in the mornings to deal with bowel evacuation. In these and other areas, such as learning how to cope with transfers and general mobility, it was generally agreed that there was a great deal one had to learn about oneself over the years. People explained how they came to understand signs such as headaches or sweating as pointing to possible problems with bladder and bowels or even skin, but one man said:

> There is so much learning to be done that nobody can teach you.

While we did not systematically collect data on pain, the problem was raised in a significant number of the interviews. Thus, one person said:

> I've recently been thinking 'how long will this go on?' Though I try to think that tomorrow you'll feel better. It's this infernal stomach pain always.

And another said:

> Life would be different if I didn't have this pain.

And a third:

> When I get pain I can't do anything and I get bored.

This pain, of unknown origin, is usually called 'root pain' and is very difficult to treat, except with pain-killers. However, one person noted the dangers of this approach:

> I have continual pain so my doctor gives me these pain-killers. They're essential, but they send me high and they're addictive. I'm not addicted but I don't see why I should go without them and have pain.

A number of people expressed concern about the prescription of such drugs, both for pain and the treatment of muscle spasms, seemingly without due regard for possible side-effects, dependence and even addiction.

As well as the possible problems of side-effects from or addiction to pain-killers, some people were angry that medical staff did not always take this pain seriously. One person had even been to a second spinal unit to have his pain investigated, but he reported:

> If for some reason it's not in the book, then you're not experiencing it. . . .
> They haven't cured it, they've tried to say it was all in my mind because the X-rays didn't show anything. But since then I've been to the general hospital and they've found something.

Clearly, then, pain, its consequences and medical treatment adversely affects the lives of many people who have spinal injuries.

CONCLUSIONS

In this chapter we have considered some of the medical aspects of spinal injury from a career perspective and identified three stages in this part of the disability career. Clearly, general hospitals are usually unable to cope with the specialist aspects of spinal injury, and this can cause unnecessary medical problems. The spinal unit was much more effective in the way it coped with the medical aspects of spinal injury, although it was criticised on the grounds of the inflexible nature of the rehabilitation process and the way people were told about their injuries. For a significant number of those interviewed, a variety of medical problems had occurred throughout their disability career after discharge from the spinal unit, although only half had maintained any regular contact with the spinal unit.

It is clear to us that while spinal injury does create considerable problems of medical management, both for professionals and for those with a spinal injury, most of these problems can be overcome by skilled intervention and long-term monitoring from a specialist spinal unit. This implies that the spinal injury service must be available throughout the disability career; from the time of injury, the person should be transferred to the spinal unit as soon as possible, he should be treated there until ready for discharge, and on discharge he should be offered regular check-ups and access to a specialist spinal bed if severe medical problems manifest themselves. This means that the spinal injuries service must be properly funded and resources to become a 'cradle to grave', or perhaps 'accident to grave', service, for, in our view, only in this way can the intrusion of medical problems into the disability career be reduced to an absolute minimum.

CHAPTER 4

Personal and Family Responses to Spinal Cord Injury

INTRODUCTION

In this chapter we shall discuss the impact that spinal injury has upon the individual and his family. The conceptual framework developed earlier will be used to discuss the data, and we shall illustrate our examples with quotations from the individuals with a spinal injury and from other family members who participated in some of the interviews as key informants. Before presenting the data, however, it is necessary to discuss further our conceptual framework and, in particular, to explain our usage of the term 'social adjustment'.

Earlier we were critical of the psychological approaches to the study of spinal cord injury on the grounds that they were over-deterministic and only considered the personal responses rather than wider social circumstances. In particular, 'stage theories' were criticised on the grounds that:

> ... evidence for such theories is either questionable, due to methodological problems; controversial as a result of vague definitions of terms; or non-existent.
>
> (Vargo and Stewin, 1984:254)

Despite this, psychological theories and stage models have also been used in studies of the families of people with spinal cord injuries (Bray, 1977, 1978; Weller and Miller, 1977). Thus, one study of 180 families with a spinally injured member suggested:

> The family of the severely disabled individual experiences many of the same emotions, concerns and conflicts as the client. They progress through developmental stages that parallel the adjustment process of the client.
>
> (Bray, 1977:237)

34

Stage models of family adjustment can be criticised on the same grounds as those of individual adjustment; that is, they are over-deterministic and too narrow in focus. Further, Cook (1976) suggests that some family reactions are attributable to the expectations and attitudes of staff rather than to any intrinsic psychological processes. Another study (Vargo and Stewin, 1984) found no evidence for the existence of these stages but found that theoretical assumptions may act as the impetus for a self-fulfilling prophecy.

Our concern is not to deny that spinal cord injury may have a profound impact on individuals and their families, but rather that existing theories and models provide an inadequate framework for describing the substantial range of responses which might occur or the wide variety of personal, social, economic and environmental factors which might be influential. That spinal cord injury is a significant life event for individuals and families there can be no doubt:

> For most people spinal cord injury demands changes in almost every aspect of life—personal relationships, the physical structure of the home, work and education, social and leisure pursuits, and financial management.
>
> (Grundy *et al.*, 1986:40)

For these reasons it is impossible to see the responses to spinal cord injury as adjustment solely in personal and family terms, but rather in the context of a much wider set of factors. Therefore, we have developed the concept of social adjustment by which we mean 'the complex relationship between the functional limitations of the person with a spinal injury, the social restrictions faced and the meanings that both these functional limitations and social restrictions have both for the individual and his family' (Creek *et al.*, 1987). This concept, alongside those of career, significant life event and meaning, will therefore be used in what follows to illuminate the wide variety of personal and family responses to spinal injury which we found in our study.

FACTORS AFFECTING PERSONAL RESPONSES

We asked all those interviewed how well they felt they coped with their disability, in terms of use of their time, the help available and equipment supplied, as well as matters relating to employment, housing and income. Thus, the question encompasses physical and material circumstances, as well as personal attitude towards managing disability in line with our concept of social adjustment. Table 4.1 shows the distribution of scores on satisfaction with disabled role for our sample. It can be seen that nearly two-thirds (62.6%) of the total sample were rated as

Table 4.1   Satisfaction with disabled role

Reaction	Number	Percentage
Satisfied	28	37.3
Minor dissatisfaction	25	33.3
Marked dissatisfaction	16	21.3
Severe dissatisfaction	6	8.0
	75	100

Missing cases = 2.

experiencing dissatisfaction at some level, with just under a third of respondents rated as being markedly or severely dissatisfied with some aspects of their disabled role.

We found three factors—age at injury, length of time since injury and current age—which were important to social adjustment.

Table 4.2 shows that the percentage of respondents expressing marked or severe dissatisfaction increased with age at the time of injury. Men who were younger at the time of injury (aged 19 or less) expressed far less marked or severe dissatisfaction than did those who received their injury later in life (aged 45 or more). Only a small number of people were aged 60 or more at the time of injury, and therefore we were unable to examine these trends beyond the age of 45, having collapsed categories 45–59/60+.

The length of time since injury was an important factor relating to social adjustment, and Table 4.3 illustrates the relationship between length of time since injury and expressed personal satisfaction. From this it can be seen that although there is little difference in expressed levels of satisfaction between the group of people injured 0–4 years and the group injured 5–9 years ago, there is a much higher percentage of people injured 10–15 years ago who expressed satisfaction with coping with their disability; 56% compared with 26% for those injured 4 years

Table 4.2   Relationship between age at time of injury and satisfaction with disabled role

Level of satisfaction	Age					Row total
	19	20–24	25–34	35–44	45+	
Satisfied (%)	42.9	52.6	15.4	14.3	40.0	37.3
Minor dissatisfaction (%)	38.1	26.3	53.8	28.6	20.0	33.3
Marked/severe dissatisfaction (%)	19.0	21.1	30.8	57.1	40.0	29.3
	100	100	100	100	100	100
	21	19	13	7	15	75

Table 4.3 Relationship between length of time since injury and satisfaction with disabled role

Level of satisfaction	Time (years)			
	0–4	*5–9*	*10–15*	*Row total*
Satisfied (%)	26.1	29.6	56.0	37.3
Minor dissatisfaction (%)	39.1	37.0	24.0	33.3
Marked/severe dissatisfaction (%)	34.8	33.3	20.0	29.3
	100	100	100	100
	23	27	25	75

Table 4.4 Relationship between age at interview and satisfaction with disabled role

Level of satisfaction	Age					
	24	*25–34*	*35–44*	*45–59*	*60+*	*Row total*
Satisfied (%)	35.7	39.3	33.3	11.1	66.7	37.3
Minor dissatisfaction (%)	35.7	39.3	33.3	44.4	0.0	33.3
Marked/severe dissatisfaction (%)	28.6	21.4	33.3	44.4	33.3	29.3
	100	100	100	100	100	100
	14	28	15	9	9	75

or less prior to interview. Those who had received their injuries within the last 4 years expressed marked or severe dissatisfaction more than those injured longer ago, but those injured between 5 and 9 years ago were nearly as likely to express serious dissatisfaction as were the recently injured group. Thus, people who had received their injury between 10 and 15 years ago were rated as satisfied far more frequently than were those injured within the last 9 years. It appears that the level of satisfaction individuals express increases with length of time since injury. An alternative interpretation poses the possibility that expression of dissatisfaction decreases with increased length of time since injury. During the first 9 years following spinal cord injury, then, our data suggest that there is likely to be some sort of dissatisfaction, albeit for the most part minor.

Finally, current age was also an important factor, and Table 4.4 shows the relationship between expressed satisfaction with disabled role and age of the person at the time of interview. Younger people were more likely to express satisfaction with their disabled role than were older people. Thus, those aged between 24 and 44 years at the time of interview expressed less dissatisfaction on this item than did men older than 45. This trend suggests that older spinally injured people experience greater dissatisfaction with their disabled role and raises important questions for subsequent research to be concerned with the ageing spinally injured population. It is of interest to note this trend in the context of expressed satisfaction seemingly increasing with length of time since injury shown by Tables 4.2 and 4.3.

We suggest two possible factors to account for increasing satisfaction over time among those interviewed. First, individual experiences of disability—personal, social and physical—are gradual. It seems that most people reach a 'plateau' of adjustment within the first 9 years. Second, there is also the possibility that the propensity to *express* dissatisfaction declines over time. In fact, these may be complementary tendencies; it is possible, therefore, that those who were injured at an older age have not had the same amount of time to adjust to changed life circumstances. Consequently, they would be more likely to express dissatisfaction at the time of interview. Their levels of satisfaction and coping with disability may subsequently increase over time, although our data do not allow for examination of this possibility.

EXTENT OF IMPAIRMENT AND PERSONAL RESPONSES

Common-sense assumptions lead to the expectation that the more severely disabled a person is—that is, the higher the lesion—the more likely he is to express dissatisfaction. However, our discussion of social adjustment suggests that a whole range of other factors have to be taken into account. Table 4.5 shows the relationship between level of lesion and the satisfaction experienced with life as a disabled person, and suggests some, but not srong, association between these two factors.

A higher percentage of those with incomplete lesions showed some

Table 4.5   Relationship between level of lesion and satisfaction with disabled role

	Level					
Level of satisfaction	*Com tetra*	*Incom tetra*	*Com para*	*Incom para*	*multi*	*Row total*
Satisfied (%)	28.6	25.0	41.7	61.5	25.0	37.3
Minor dissatisfaction (%)	57.1	25.0	33.3	15.4	50.0	33.3
Marked/severe dissatisfaction (%)	14.3	50.0	25.0	23.1	25.0	29.3
	100	100	100	100	100	100
	14	20	24	13	4	75

signs of dissatisfaction than did people with complete lesions. A possible explanation may consist in the marginality of this particular group, being neither completely disabled nor completely able-bodied. Only slight differences in expressed levels of dissatisfaction were found between people with complete lesions, suggesting that extent of impairment is not a significant factor in social adjustment. However, as later chapters will show, the relationship between satisfaction with disability (social adjustment) and time is not a simple one but is related to a whole range of other factors, material and social. Whether it is possible to return to work; how suitable housing is and how long it takes to obtain it; levels of income, which may change over time; the delays in compensation settlements; and so on: these are all factors which make time a crucial component of social adjustment. It is not a matter of 'time being a great healer', but of the speed (or lack of it) with which support services are mobilised, as well as changing perceptions and relationships that occur throughout the disability career. Each of these factors may be different for each individual, so social adjustment is not about following a path through fixed stages but rather about negotiating a passage through the disability career.

The material presented above provides a useful framework for discussion of personal responses to spinal cord injury. However, exploring these sorts of issues is very complicated. There are important individual differences, for example, not only in age, length of time since injury, and level and type of lesion, but also in physical, psychological and social factors, and therefore in personal responses. Qualitative material, in the form of extracts from interviews, enables deeper exploration of the issue of personal response to spinal cord injury and will be heavily drawn on throughout the rest of this chapter. As in other chapters, we shall attempt to present this material from the 'disability career' perspective and to look at personal responses of injured persons and their family members over time. We shall focus principally on three stages in the disability career: the time of the injury, discharge and the immediate post-discharge period, and the present.

PERSONAL RESPONSES AT THE TIME OF INJURY

In accordance with the finding that length of time since injury is related to expressed satisfaction after injury, people we interviewed often said that the process of getting used to what had happened to them had taken time. Some men explained that when first told the nature of their injury, they had felt too ill to take it in properly or to fully appreciate what they were being told, saying, for example, 'It didn't really sink in. I thought it was a bad dream'.

Several people felt that they had resisted hearing what they were being told, and described how at first they had refused to believe it. One man recalled:

> I just didn't believe it. It took a month of total disbelief. They told me and I thought, 'I don't believe you, I'm afraid'. You don't really want to accept it.

For some people this was a fairly short-lived phase of coming to terms with what had happened to them, whereas for others it took much longer to work through initial trauma and shock. Six months after injury was frequently described as the period before which people began to respond to what had happened to them in any realistic or constructive sense: 'It took 6 months for me to be able to face up to anything'. Most of those injured said they had realised what had happened much sooner than this—saying, for example, 'I just knew straight away', or said that after a week or two they clearly understood what had happened, but this was not necessarily the point at which they had begun to respond to their injury.

Of course, initial responses to spinal cord injury varied a great deal. One person claimed:

> I just faced up to it. I didn't have dark images or anything. I just thought, 'OK. This has happened. Let's get on and live.'

However, it was not uncommon for respondents to remark that at first they had felt depressed:

> When I realised what my life was going to be like I felt pretty pissed off.

One went so far as to say:

> At the time I thought it was the end of the world.

One person said:

> When you've walked all your life and you think you'll never walk again . . . it's difficult to explain . . . it's just one big shock.

Relatives, as well as the injured person, found the initial phase of responding to what had happened difficult. The impact of the spinal cord injury was sometimes more profound for relatives at this stage than for the injured person. One injured person explained that:

> . . . because of so much happening in a relatively short space of time, it probably had far more impact on the people who were around me than myself.

A conversation that took place during one of the interviews between the injured person and his wife describes this further. The husband said:

> I think it's such a massive thing that you can't actually take it in to start with, can you? My wife was very shocked and numbed by it because she could probably understand it more clearly than I could.

His wife explained her perspective at the time, saying:

> Well . . . as he [the doctor] was saying 'your husband is going to be totally paralysed' . . . I just had this bird's eye view of my whole future where I saw me just pushing you around, doing everything for you, and actually I just thought well . . . right . . . I'll do it. I mean it would have been far worse if you had died, you see, that was the thing I didn't want to happen. When I thought of pushing you around in a wheelchair and doing everything for you I didn't know what it entailed, and I didn't know all the grind, but I thought well, I'll do anything for him.

Relatives described their additional trauma of handling the immediate responses of loved ones on first learning the nature of their injury. The accounts of relatives vividly reflect the shock and difficulties experienced by the injured person in the very first stages of facing up to it. The wife of one injured man explained during an interview:

> I can remember sitting in Stoke Mandeville and he was lying there and he said 'Do you think anything much about me?' and I said 'Yes' . . . and he said, 'If you think anything about me, give me something, finish it for me.' He said, 'I would rather you finished it for me now.' And I can remember thinking yes, and I think I would want that too if I was laying there. But in no way could I . . . but by God . . . and I talked to every man in that ward while I was there, month after month after month, and there wasn't a man there that didn't wish he'd died.

In the majority of cases, however, members of the injured person's family, on whom so much stress devolved, remained unsupported by staff in the hospital, or professionals from outside. Several people commented that the role taken on by relatives in the hospital needed to be recognised.

Many relatives recalled the shock of learning the nature of the injury and both their sense of isolation and the lack of support they felt they had received from the spinal unit staff. There was particular resentment voiced at the lack of opportunity to discuss the injury with the doctors involved in their relatives' treatment, although a few relatives of people most recently injured did praise the help and time given by junior doctors. Distance and difficulties of visiting other than at weekends sometimes compounded this problem, particularly as Stoke Mandeville has a much larger catchment area than have the other spinal units. It was usually also true that at this stage community support services had not been mobilised and, thus, relatives often had no support at all, from either the hospital or community-based professionals.

PERSONAL RESPONSES ON DISCHARGE FROM HOSPITAL

Discharge from hospital was also recalled as a critical time in personal response to injury: critical for ex-patient and family. Several people described how they had begun to feel more positive and optimistic as discharge from hospital became imminent, although this was also a time of anxiety. One person encapsulated both these positive and negative aspects:

> You have fear when you come out of Stoke Mandeville ... there was a fear, but not a fear that would deter you from trying. I thought—you've got two choices—either you adapt yourself to being in a wheelchair and get on with it, or you give up. You've just got to get on with it.

Leaving hospital was sometimes a difficult experience on top of the problems of learning to live with the physical consequences of the spinal injury. Many people said that they had been nervous about leaving hospital and some acknowledged that this had made them touchy and irritable for a while. Returning home and fitting back into family life was not always easy after long periods of being in hospital. The comments of one man describe an experience of first going home:

> It was a pretty churning experience really because I was desperately looking forward to being home with my lovely wife and family. I got there and found that I couldn't manoeuvre the wheelchair out of the house. The children were always shouting, whereas in the hospital if you wanted to be quiet, you could wheel yourself off into a corner and be quiet. I found I got very tired and couldn't necessarily relax and go to bed whenever I wanted to at home, whereas in hospital there was much more of a routine and you tended to have your days planned so that when you were tired you could go to bed sort of thing. No, it's very strange. At the time I felt very weird—totally torn really between wanting to be home with the family and being there with the family and finding that I was coping very badly. You know, you get all crabby and bad-tempered and pretty tired and the children don't behave like clockwork, they behave like children.

After discharge from hospital some people described periods of weakness or poor health. Many men spoke of physical strain over the first few months after returning home, and, for some, physical problems continued or recurred indefinitely. In terms of personal responses, initial health problems often coincided with periods of depression, lethargy, irritability and loss of confidence. Leaving hospital was described as an anticlimax in relation to a 'high' that several people experienced in hospital, particularly on first getting out of bed:

> When I came out [of hospital] I had that sort of down phase. It wasn't for very long . . . the wife did a lot of work on me. She said 'don't be so bloody silly' or words to that effect, but you do. It's indescribable really . . . you feel that everything's down about you. That was soon afterwards. I was trying to do things that at that time were physically impossible and it really did get me down.

One man gave the following retrospective interpretation of depression he experienced shortly after leaving hospital:

> It was funny really, but for a long time I just didn't realise that of course I was going through a stressful time, and that of course I was going to find difficulty adjusting to it, and that of course that was why I was depressed . . . I needed somebody to say to me 'Look, *this* is *why* you are depressed. You've got to pick yourself up and start a new life.'

For some, optimism fostered in the protective hospital environment precipitated an emotional crash on discharge. Another man explained:

> I didn't realise when I was in Stoke Mandeville, how depressing it would be coming home. I don't think that most people realise how the memories suddenly come flooding back. You're very protected in hospital.

Several people felt strongly that they and their families had not been adequately prepared for coming to terms with their disability after hospital:

> It's another world in Stoke Mandeville. It's different when you come out.

This could be particularly true for those who did not go back to where they had been living prior to injury, or to live with their family. For people in these circumstances, many factors relating to the issue of where they want to live after discharge from hospital obviously had important ramifications for personal response to spinal cord injury. One man, for example, described his feelings about moving to live in a unit for young disabled people after discharge:

> When I got there I thought, 'God. I'm 30. I've got a bed and a box of things.' I stared out of the window. I turned to the bottle. I closed my eyes and burst into tears. I thought *panic*.

Problems could be encountered in personal and family relationships during the early homecoming period. Despite the great appreciation for the help often received from relatives, family support sometimes presented a mixed blessing. Twenty-eight people were living with parents at the time of the accident, and a number who had previously been living away from home, returned to parents on discharge from hospital. Some praised their parents' attitudes:

> The great thing is they have still given me my freedom as well as being really supportive.

Others spoke of acute difficulties in the first few months after leaving hospital coping with over-protective parents, when they themselves were struggling to be independent:

> It was terrible . . . awful. I was independent before my accident and they were very good to me but they treated me as if I was 6 years old and I needed my independence.

This was also the case for some people living away from home but was more often a problem for those living at home; being in the same household could give rise to a period of severe confrontation lasting, in some cases, up to a year or more. One man, for example, related:

> Ultimately . . . I told her [my mother] that I was going to kill myself if she carried on. I mean literally . . . and that shocked her into changing her attitude towards me . . . she really treated me like a baby. I had to say something, otherwise our relationship would have continued to be more and more damaged.

Sometimes, but not always, these initial strains were said to have been resolved into a deeper and happier relationship, with parents recognising the needs of the individual with spinal cord injury and their own abilities:

> On discharge, my mother was very worried about doing the right thing for fear of any more injury but now she realises that she doesn't need to be so careful, she realises her capabilities and how far she can go.

Often relatives acknowledged their difficulties in responding appropriately to the spinally injured person when first discharged. The wife of one man explained:

> For the first 5 years I never left him at all because . . . if you've been to hospital for about 9 months . . . I remember thinking 'I don't want him to go back again' . . . so you make yourself a martyr and you never leave him for about 5 years.

And those injured recognise that at the time they could not always make a positive contribution to important relationships. One man revealed:

> I was suffering from the problems of trying to readjust from the accident and I was not being particularly helpful at that stage. Anyone who got in the way was soaking up the abuse which was fairly evil but it was a period I had to go through.

Many people reiterated the thoughts of one man who said:

> On discharge it was difficult to cope and get back to a family life-style. You have to relearn to live with other people again.

A few people mentioned ways in which spinal injury affected relationships with children or with brothers and sisters. Sometimes these relationships were adversely affected, as in the case of one man who was saddened because his eldest son found seeing his father in a wheelchair traumatic and subsequently preferred not to visit. The wife of another injured man told us that their teenage daughter had wanted to go to boarding school after her father's accident and went on to say:

> She loved it. All the other girls used to cry when they went back to school, and she was happy as a sandboy, and the other mothers used to say, 'What did you say to her? How do you do it?' And I thought 'if only they knew', I felt like crying; she wanted to go away.

In the great majority of families, however, relationships were not said to have deteriorated since a person's spinal injury, and often new dimensions came to relationships such as greater closeness between brothers and sisters, fathers and daughters, mothers and sons.

PERSONAL RESPONSES OVER TIME

The length of time involved in the process of getting used to having a spinal cord injury was emphasised by many of those interviewed, and their relatives:

> The trouble is that it *does* take a long time to get used to it—not that I couldn't accept it. I mean I knew I wasn't going to walk again, and God knows how many years until this operation comes along and they'll be able to do something about it . . . I knew I was going to be in that chair for the rest of my life and I still do—unless some miracle occurs. After about 3 years I was used to it.

One man said:

> I found everybody has the same experience, it does take *years* before
> things suddenly click into place and you are going to be certainly suffering
> physically and *mentally* for a very long time, long after you leave hospital,
> and it can take anything, as I gather listening to other people, anything
> between 2 years and 6 years perhaps, and then things suddenly do fall
> into place and life goes on fairly normally.

It would appear from these comments that adjustment is often
thought of as a continuous process, with the time factor being a crucial
dimension. This reflects our earlier suggestion that length of time since
injury is important. People who had been injured less than 10 years
prior to interview tended to speak more cogently of ongoing difficulties
and coming to terms with their disability than did others, and expressed
greater dissatisfaction and more problems coping. The comments of
some respondents interviewed within a few years of having received
their injury vividly portray the depression that occurred for some in the
early stages of response to injury:

> I haven't got a normal life, you know. I'm not particularly happy but I've
> got used to it . . . to a certain degree . . . I feel sometimes I'm treading on a
> knife's edge as far as my nerves are concerned—you know it really is bad.
> I thought one time I was going to have a nervous breakdown or
> something, it got really chronic . . . not being able to cope with it I
> suppose. I probably will go right over the edge . . . have a breakdown of
> some description. I cope, but it's just about like. It's all nervous strain, it's
> like an intense fear. I don't really know what I'm scared of, it's such a
> peculiar thing. I never used to be like it. It's just since the accident.

Another man recently out of hospital said:

> I feel terrible, I can't think. It's happened and there's nothing you can do.
> You've still got your arms and your head, you can still get around with the
> wheels . . . but I find it very hard. Sometimes I have to put a tape on to get
> things off my mind about this lot.

Several of those interviewed described an initial period of almost
obsessive enthusiasm to fill time by trying to improve fitness after first
leaving hospital, and commitment to exercise was clearly in itself
energising for some people in the early stages. One man said:

> When I first came home it was mainly exercise, standing and weights until
> the end of the afternoon and then tea. In the evening I used to go to the
> therapy pool. My main concern was to keep fit and healthy. My time was
> occupied by trying to keep healthy. It was all physical.

Thus far we have attempted to present an overview of the range of personal responses encountered by those injured and their relatives, in order to portray something of the considerable variance in personal response to spinal cord injury among the men interviewed as part of this research.

The process of personal and family response to spinal injury also has a crucial time element in it, and it is not just a matter of going through a series of stages in the immediate aftermath of the injury. Nor is adjustment ever completed, for social adjustment is a continuous process throughout the life-cycle and involves a complex interplay of personal, family, social and material factors. As one man put it:

> The first thing to do is survive. Then once you've achieved survival you can start putting the gloss on.

This statement reflects the experience of many of those interviewed, reiterating the finding that length of time since injury is an important factor in personal response. However, response to spinal injury is enormously influenced by individual differences. Some of those interviewed responded to their spinal injury very differently compared with others, and social adjustment is never complete, for, as another put it:

> I have spent half my life in a wheelchair. I don't know how I've been affected. I just know that I'm not over the moon about it. Life is what you make it. I'm reasonably happy, but I'm not over the moon about it. I let life carry on. I take it as it comes.

FAMILY AND PERSONAL RELATIONSHIPS

This chapter would not be complete without some discussion of the impact of spinal cord injury on family and personal relations and the changes that may be brought about.

> The onset of severe disability can have profound effects, not necessarily damaging, on existing personal relationships and on the formation of new relationships. Disability will change the roles people undertake in a relationship: for instance, a wife whose husband is disabled may find she has to manage the family's financial and business affairs for the first time ... the able-bodied person—husband, wife or parent—may have to provide intimate personal care. The workload of everyone concerned is likely to be much greater. For many couples an active and satisfying sexual relationship may be possible, but it will be different. These changes, in addition to the feelings engendered by loss of function and its actual cause, are likely to have major repercussions.
>
> (Grundy *et al.*, 1986:40)

This, then, encapsulates some of the major issues which we will now discuss.

If we consider marital relationships first, the evidence as to whether couples where one partner has a spinal injury are more prone to break-up and divorce, is conflicting. Some have suggested that there is little difference between these couples where a spinal injury is present and those where it is not (Guttmann, 1964), while others have suggested that there is more likelihood of break-up, at least within the first 3 years (DeVivo and Fine, 1985). There are major problems in interpreting this evidence due to cultural differences, changes in family life in society generally and the different methodologies used. We do not propose to enter this controversy, although from our, albeit small, sample there is no evidence to suggest a greater likelihood of marital break-up when the husband has a spinal injury.

Twenty-six men interviewed were living with their wives when they sustained their injuries, 20 of them with children. By the time of the interview, five men from this group had been divorced and one separated, and one man had a further failed marriage and remarried his first wife. Another had remarried but subsequently separated and was in the process of divorce again. These figures would not support assumptions which are common among unit staff that there is a high incidence of divorce among spinally injured men. Where divorce did occur, it was often within a short period after the injury. Thus, in one man's case:

> I came home and the wife cleared off . . . because of the sex side of it she cleared off. I mean there is no sex and she couldn't accept that sort of thing.

Marital relationships were sometimes, although by no means invariably, altered where one partner became spinally injured. Sometimes marriages were enhanced, as, for example, one man found:

> I find this extraordinary, but I mean she [my wife] told me that she sees me as just the same person. You know she sees me as a person rather than a disabled body. And the children . . . they say, 'Oh, we don't mind . . . it doesn't really matter much does it?' Extraordinary really, but they seem to be just glad that I'm around and that I'm me . . . and I'm more friends with them now than I was before [the accident] because I've slowed down a bit and I suppose I take a bit more time and trouble with them.

Sometimes there had been some problems with the marriage prior to the injury. However, this was not always the case. One happily married man described how after discharge from hospital difficulties relating to his injury proved insurmountable:

> Things got too tough at home with my wife taking care of me and the two kids, it just got too much for her. I saw the effect it was having on her. It was dragging her down and I decided—we both decided—it had to finish.

The decision, this man said, was not difficult to arrive at but 'a bit of a killer' when put into practice. He said:

> There was nothing wrong between us. It was just the accident that caused everything to go wrong. It was inevitable.

Other couples experienced the reverse situation, whereby their marriage, collapsing at the time of the husband's accident, was salvaged because of his injury. In one such case the wife spoke bitterly of her situation, both at the time of her husband's injury and currently. She described what had happened as follows:

> At the time of the accident I thought it was the end of our marriage. Why, I wasn't at home ... our relationship was very tense. They couldn't find me to tell me about the accident. Why? Because I was at the estate agents. I was putting the house on the market. They didn't know that at the hospital. I tell them I was at work. You don't tell everyone things like that. And then it was my duty to stand by him and pick up the pieces. I blame him for his accident. I can't forgive him. The night he fell down I wasn't at home because I'd walked out. He was drinking. We were arguing. I'd just come from work. I went to sleep at a friend's house ... so I blame him in my mind ... if he hadn't been drinking he wouldn't have fallen down. I think he is at fault. I don't have the guts to say to the social services ... 'Look, I can't take any more. Take care of him.' Sometimes I want to. He's no angel. This April I went to a solicitor. Very seriously. But I believe 'in sickness and in health, 'til death us do part'. I'm obligated. I couldn't live with my conscience if I severed the relationship. But I don't know how long I can continue. I couldn't leave because of my family. We say if somebody's down you don't kick them. But our marriage is finished socially, sexually, psychologically—in every way.

A small number of women said that they felt 'trapped', by family and societal expectations, into caring for a severely disabled husband who, in other circumstances, they would have divorced long ago.

The idea that the spinal cord injury brings about a change in other personal relationships was discussed by several respondents, and was considered by some to be prohibitive in the development of new relationships. One person said:

> If the woman is *looking after you* she's always looking for something to do to you. That's the experience I've had anyway, and also of relationships I've seen with other disabled people and it's always looked rather unattractive—the woman sort of doing it all. So I think to myself, 'Yeah, well I do want to be married, but I don't want to be married like that.'

Another man's feelings were similar:

> This disability is too big to consider a relationship. If you're having a relationship with someone you've got to be convinced you're giving as much as taking. With people like me there's too much taking.

Some felt their disability presented an obstacle to relationships with women, and reservations in this respect were expressed by several men, summarised by one person thus:

> I could probably do more to make opportunities, but the disability is a barrier. It bugs me. It makes me feel inferior to most men. I don't know if the problem is really in my own head. It might be. It's after making the first contact . . . carrying it on to be more than that. I find the disability restricting psychologically. It's so difficult to break the ice. I feel that people shy away from close contact with disabled people. Relationships don't carry on to the same extent that they might have.

Several men reported loss of self-confidence for personal relationships, often associated with embarrassment about physique, or anxiety about the shape or condition of their body:

> You've got to believe in yourself before someone else can believe in you, and I don't. I haven't got confidence. I think anyone would be put off. I'm embarrassed about the shape of my body and the way I look.

Many worries were expressed about sexuality, and dissatisfaction with sexual function. One respondent told us:

> At first, all I could think of was sex.

The comments of those injured as young men did support this suggestion:

> The sexual side does bother me. It's the worst thing about being in a wheelchair. It does you in mentally.

Another person said:

> It's the sex side you think about more than anything.

Many people made similar remarks.

Sex was considered to be an important factor for many people. One older man said:

> At my age it's the family relationship rather than sexual that is of major

importance. Not that sex is unimportant, but it's not the overriding concern.

Several people shared the view of another man, who said:

I've put sex and relationships right out of my mind.

A range of explanations were given as to why this should be so, of which the following is fairly typical:

When a man's disabled like I am, sex is all too awkward and it wouldn't make me happy at all and I can't see why any woman would want to cope with it anyway. I really can't understand why a woman would want to put herself up for a thing like that.

For a few spinally injured men, dependent on personal care, intimate relationships were explicitly rejected, because they felt the introduction of a partner into the household, or developing a relationship with those providing this personal care, would potentially disrupt their physical and/or emotional well-being. During the research it became obvious that the implications of change in sexual function did not comprise part of the rehabilitation for most people in our study, and many criticisms have been made of this. We were told of a range of similarly inadequate communications on the subject, from 'the whole subject wasn't ever mentioned' to 'we had a couple of diagrams and were told: "Your sex life's finished".' These are critical issues, given the importance of sex and sexuality in many personal relationships.

Another especially difficult experience for several people had been seeing negative effects of their injury upon other members of the family. Several men expressed concern about the strain imposed on parents who were caring for them, and said that this often gave rise to feelings of guilt and conflict. In one man's experience, for example:

I feel I put so much on my dad. I do as much as I can but it's not much . . . I feel guilty about how much I put on him. Sometimes I get frustrated and lash out at him. It's not him, it's myself—always depending on him. I don't like him to have to do everything for me especially now he is older. We argue about stupid things. I end up swearing at him, it upsets him and it upsets me. I feel guilty. I don't mean it.

These worries were often compounded by fears for the future. One man who lived with his mother and younger brothers and sisters, spoke about such concerns:

Obviously I'm extra responsibility. At times it does . . . not upset me, but worry me. Because she has to work all day and I know that she's got to come in from work and do something about me. And I think ... well, any other woman who works all day can just come in and sit down and have a cup of tea and that'll be it. But she's got to worry about what she's got to do with me that night. I mean she doesn't get up from watching the telly and go straight to bed. She's got to get up from watching the telly, come in and put me to bed, and then go to bed and she can't sleep well because she's got one ear open in case I need her and shout to her in the night. Yeah, it does worry me a lot. Especially if she's not feeling well. Then I think I'm a burden. It does worry me. And if something happened to her, what would happen to the family?

Relatives also voiced concern about their long-term ability to sustain their role as principal providers of care. As we have pointed out elsewhere, this care had physical and emotional consequences for the relatives. Thus, the wife of a tetraplegic man stated:

Let me put it this way: if I could live my life again I'd say 'No'. I wouldn't have one day of it. That's how much of a strain it is looking after somebody.

Furthermore, just as many of those with spinal injuries expressed concern about the consequences of ageing, many relatives were concerned that as they grew older they would no longer be able to cope with the demands of looking after tetraplegics in particular. So one mother who looked after her tetraplegic son commented:

We are getting older and it does become harder getting up in the night, losing sleep ... especially for my husband with work the next day.

These anxieties and stresses were not only apparent in the families of tetraplegics, however; within other families, adults and sometimes older children also reported feeling the burden of responsibility for looking after someone else. For a few, these responsibilities were felt, regardless of extent of disability or the need for assistance. Thus, the wife of an incomplete paraplegic who was ambulant commented:

I worry about how you would manage without us.

In some families these concerns had been openly discussed, and occasionally plans had been made with the family to cope with such contingencies as illness, ageing or death of the carer. Other families acknowledged that this might become a problem but plans had not yet been formulated. Thus, the wife of a paraplegic noted:

I suppose as long as I keep reasonably fit then there is no problem but if something happened to me then there might be a problem ... we just hope the the social services will rally round ....

In the meanwhile respite care offered considerable sustenance for some of those caring for spinally injured people. The physical and emotional implications of the caring situation meant that relatives sometimes needed, and the disabled person required, a break. Many families were not able to arrange respite care. The SIA Care Attendant Scheme had been used by some families, but many did not know about the scheme, or were apprehensive about using it. However, anxieties about respite care provision can be readily understood from the experience of one elderly woman, caring for her severely disabled husband, who on the advice of her own GP had arranged with her husband a short stay in a local hospital. On arrival:

> . . . the sister on the ward said to him, 'My ward could be full of holiday people like you. I don't see why I should have you', . . . and he just sort of sat there and cringed, and he said he sat there and thought, 'Oh I wish the ground would swallow me up'. So you see he won't go again.

Standards of respite care had been found unacceptable by several families, a finding which has been documented before (Briggs and Oliver, 1984).

Households including a paid care attendant reported the least dissatisfaction, whereas households comprising a married couple registered the most dissatisfaction. It is likely that this finding relates to the difficulties illustrated above, which arise when, following her husband's spinal cord injury, the nature of the marital relationship changes to the extent that the wife comes to function predominantly as care attentant (Oliver, 1984). The quality of household relationships will obviously be a major determinant of satisfaction with one's life. In accordance with this, we found that spinally injured people living with friends reported less dissatisfaction than did those living with family members, either parents or spouse.

The fact that our data suggest that people are more satisfied when living with care attendants or friends rather than family is clearly important, but it should be rememberd that the actual numbers living in this way are small. What may be important about this is the issue of choice; many of those we interviewed, and indeed their families, felt that the decision to return to the family home was not a matter of choice at all. Rather it was based on the assumption of professionals that the family situation was the appropriate place to which to return the person with a spinal injury, and was constrained by the fact that no acceptable alternatives were available. On the other hand, those living with friends or care attendants had chosen so to do. The implications of this for rehabilitation and service provision are obvious and do not need to be spelt out here.

CONCLUSIONS

Social adjustment to spinal cord injury is not, therefore, a unidimensional problem, as the stage theorists would have it, but a multidimensional one. The process of social adjustment comprises a series of interactions between individuals and their physical and social environments, and is mediated by the meanings these interactions have for these individuals and their families. Obviously, there are differences in people's objective circumstances and this may make it easier for some than others, but it is clear that individual differences in the way people subjectively experience spinal cord injury are also profoundly important. However, we would not like to give the impression that, because the process of social adjustment is unique to each individual, no planned and systematic programme of support can be provided.

Most importantly, length of time since injury is associated with social adjustment, and, in part, this is a reflection of the length of time that people take to amass sufficient personal, social and economic resources in order to be able to cope. Throughout the disability career, the support necessary for social adjustment is lacking: counselling, of both the individual and his family, was inadequate in the early stages after injury; there was little or no continuity of support after discharge; and the provision of services was usually slow, bureaucratic and unnecessarily harrowing. If these conditions were significantly improved, then the process of social adjustment might not take 9 years, as it appears to at present, and much unnecessary suffering could be relieved for all concerned.

CHAPTER 5

Leisure, Social Life and Mobility in the Community

INTRODUCTION

In this chapter we shall consider some of the restrictions on social and leisure activities experienced on return to the community. We shall also describe various ways in which people adapted to these restrictions over time. In keeping with our conceptual framework of the disability career, the main focus will be on the changes people had made in their social and leisure activities, and their changing perceptions of this area of their lives.

The effects of restrictions on personal mobility will also be discussed in some detail. Several previous studies have shown that much of our environment—particularly in urban areas—is inaccessible even to people with only minor physical impairments (Barker and Bury, 1978; Buchanan and Chamberlain, 1978; Denby et al., 1978). Furthermore, the inaccessibility of the environment is often exacerbated by people with physical impairments being handicapped in their use of transport (GLAD, 1986). For example, a recent study of transport use by young disabled people found that over 75% of the sample were completely unable to use the public transport system (Hoad, 1986). Consequently, many were reliant on the availability of private transport for their mobility. Indeed, this and other studies cited here have highlighted the importance of transport and mobility for disabled people being able to enjoy satisfactory social lives. Conversely, lack of adequate transport and other restrictions on mobility can lead to social isolation and a marked curtailment of leisure activities (Jowett, 1982; Rowan, 1979).

We shall start this chapter by considering the factors which influenced levels of people's satisfaction with their leisure activities. The discussion will then be broadened out to consider the development of people's social lives and personal relationships after injury. Finally, we shall examine the important effects of restrictions on mobility on these areas of their lives.

LEISURE TIME AND ACTIVITIES

The analysis of our interview data confirms the findings of these earlier studies. Of the people we interviewed, 90% had some restriction on their opportunities for leisure and over 50% had marked or severe restrictions (Creek *et al.*, 1987: 127). In terms of the subjective meaning individuals attached to the quality of their leisure activities, however, we found a significant contrast between opportunities for, and satisfaction with, leisure. Table 5.1 shows that nearly half of the people we interviewed were satisfied with their leisure, and less than 20% expressed significant levels of dissatisfaction. These contrasting findings suggest that satisfaction with leisure activities is more closely related to the opportunities which individuals perceive to be available than to the actual restrictions they encountered. Not surprisingly, individuals who

Table 5.1   Satisfaction with social contacts and leisure activities

Level of satisfaction	Social contacts	Leisure activities
Satisfied (%)	52.6	44.2
Minor dissatisfaction (%)	30.3	36.4
Marked dissatisfaction (%)	10.5	11.7
Severe dissatisfaction (%)	6.6	7.8
	100.0	100.0
Base totals	(76)	(77)

perceived their opportunities for leisure activities to be adequate, or nearly so, were most likely to express satisfaction. However, a significant minority who perceived their opportunities for leisure activities to be markedly or severely inadequate still expressed satisfaction or only minor dissatisfaction. As we shall illustrate below, the contrast between opportunities for, and satisfaction with, leisure activities reflects the tendency for people to adjust to their changed circumstances over time. Indeed, the ability to develop new interests was a significant and positive aspect of the disability career for many of the people we interviewed.

The variations in levels of satisfaction and dissatisfaction also suggest that marked or severe restrictions on opportunities for leisure may be 'compensated' for by other factors which influence satisfaction. In terms of expressed satisfaction with leisure, statistical analysis revealed that level of lesion, employment status and car ownership were particularly significant.

Paraplegics were significantly more satisfied with their leisure than were tetraplegics (see Creek *et al.*, 1987:130). The range of leisure activities open to individuals with higher-level lesions is more restricted than for those with lesser degrees of impairment. For example, many people reported having previously enjoyed sporting and other physical activities; continuation of such physical activities often proved easier for paraplegics than for people with lesions of very high level.

There were also other physically related problems which were experienced by people with both lower- and higher-level lesions. Visiting other people in their own homes, for example, presented many people with difficulties. These difficulties primarily concerned access, but such matters as heating levels and dietary requirements also posed problems for some individuals:

> I do feel embarrassed if I go to someone's home and I keep my coat on and they are all in their shirt sleeves.

> I far less look forward to going out to other people's houses—the other thing is I don't have much of an appetite so the thought of going to other people's homes and not wanting to eat much and worrying about it . . . that reduces your social life quite a bit.

Similarly, several individuals said that they found it very embarrassing and difficult to tell people (even those they knew very well) about their physical needs, such as emptying a leg bag. Indeed, the problems associated with bladder and bowel functions after spinal cord injury were reported by many as causing restrictions to their leisure activities.

Whether or not people found these physical consequences of spinal cord injury inhibiting, many felt that the lack of spontaneity in their lives following injury was a significant restriction on their social and leisure activities:

> That's the main differences—having to plan . . . everything is preplanned even down to your bowels being open . . . .

> Living life in a strict routine affects what you can do socially—[it] affects relationships and available spare time.

> You can't have such a care-free life-style.

Difficulty in actually getting out to enjoy leisure activities was also an important factor in restricting some people's satisfaction with their leisure. Several pointed to the necessity of relying on others to drive them as a further inhibiting factor in the level of spontaneity with which they could enjoy their leisure activities.

A number of people also spoke of the difficulties they had on return from hospital before they had transport of their own. This situation was often heightened by problems of access into and out of their own houses while waiting for adaptations, problems which remained for many tetraplegics. A few individuals with high-level lesions also noted the problems of dependence on carers being present for them to be able to enjoy certain leisure activities, especially out of the house. Thus, the availability of transport and independence in mobility were obviously very important factors in being able to follow satisfying leisure pursuits. This aspect of people's lives will be discussed in more detail below.

Employment was also an important factor associated with levels of expressed satisfaction with leisure activities (see Creek *et al.*, 1987:132). The majority of people who were not working felt that they had too much leisure time and insufficient meaningful and enjoyable activity to fill it—hence their higher levels of dissatisfaction. However, this was not true for everybody. For those who had been unemployed prior to their accidents and had been used to this situation, lack of employment presented fewer problems as regards opportunities for leisure. On the other hand, lack of money often placed restrictions on the range of leisure time activities which people were able to follow.

The small number of people working part-time reported a higher degree of dissatisfaction with their leisure activities than did those in full-time employment. Possibly this has something to do with the nature of the part-time work. Sometimes people were working from home, which meant there could be a lack of social contacts; also, sometimes the work was perhaps not as stimulating as some full-time jobs.

People who were in full-time employment often experienced problems balancing time between work, leisure pursuits and self-care.

> The trouble is you don't have time for most of these things if you are busy working . . . .

> . . . one of the things that I have come to realise is that if I am going to live the way that I have chosen to live and organise the care and support system and continue to negotiate with the social services to refine it and to tackle things like sorting out the day to day necessities that are involved in it, . . . it's very time-consuming and to work full-time and have some sort of continuity in maintaining social relationships, there isn't the time available—I don't have the energy.

There were many other kinds of restrictions to leisure activities noted by people we interviewed. Lack of access to buildings (private and public) and the increasing stringency of fire regulations at such places as cinemas were factors reported as restricting leisure pursuits by nearly everyone. Many people did not like being manhandled in their wheelchairs and therefore did not wish to go anywhere where they could not manage entirely by themselves:

> If somebody actually picked you up and put you down, you would hate it and yet people do not realise that you do dislike it. . . . It was one of the

few friction areas with my wife ... and there are still friends who you really have got to fight them off and almost be rude to tell them to go away. ... The rule is so simple: if I need help, I will ask and if I don't ask for it, don't push it.

Many people also mentioned that the lack of suitable access in many public places also created problems in travelling to 'unknown' territory. Consequently, they chose to stick to tried and tested areas and places. This was particularly noted in relation to holidays, where the various problems outlined above could stop even the most active from taking holidays or visiting friends and family if overnight stops were required.

I don't go on holiday because outside of this environment I hit brick walls ... you immediately hit things you can't do because of your disability ... it's at that point when you get stopped that you suddenly realise you're in a wheelchair, up to that point you don't notice it.

On their return home, many people we interviewed referred to changing leisure interests or developing leisure interests other than those they had prior to their injury. For most people, this was a gradual process, which involved changing expectations as well as finding new interests and occupations. There was also a tendency for marked or severe dissatisfaction to decrease with length of time since injury (Creek *et al.*, 1987:142). This reflects the fact that it is the meanings which individuals attach to their activities rather than the restrictions they face which is most influential in determining levels of satisfaction.

Many people mentioned missing previously enjoyed sporting or outdoor activities. For many, these very physical activities had been their major leisure pursuit prior to injury. (For some, the same activities were the cause of their accident.) Consequently, the inability to pursue previously enjoyed sports was often a significant source of frustration. Others accepted that they could no longer carry out such physical activities, or explained that, as they were growing older and as their friends grew older, they slowly gave up such activities anyway and turned to other sources of enjoyment.

However, many people had taken up new sporting activities after their injuries. Indeed, such activities were actively encouraged by staff at the spinal unit as part of the rehabilitation process. Basket-ball, archery and swimming were the most common sports that people had taken up after their injuries, although a whole range of other sports were also mentioned. Several people had developed their interests and abilities in these sports to such an extent that they had been invited to take part in the paraplegic games abroad. While most had taken up new sporting interests, a few had developed their previous activities and had become involved in the able-bodied, as well as the physically disabled, teaching and competition worlds. One man, for example, had become a fully qualified tennis coach since his injury.

A number of individuals had also decided to take some time out of their employment or education to take part in one of the various walking programmes. Nearly all of these individuals also commented on how much they now appreciated their leisure time and being able to become involved in sports again. Many people taking part in walking programmes had done so in part because of a desire to improve the image of themselves which they believed they projected to other people. It is not surprising, therefore, that sport also figured prominently in their lives.

On the other hand, there were a number of people who did not wish to take part in sports or other activities organised exclusively for disabled participants, but preferred to join in with able-bodied people for their leisure.

> Oh no, I don't want to go to the cripples' swimming club. I mean, I have a great deal of respect for the people who do go and the other people who help them but you could look at me and say: 'Poor fellow'. I could look at somebody in a wheelchair and say: 'Poor fellow' because he is as different from me as you consider me to be from you.

Among the other leisure interests people enjoyed were watching television, listening to the radio and to music, and the theatre; these were frequently interests that they had developed since their injury.

> Theatre I thoroughly enjoy. If anything my enjoyment of the theatre is probably enhanced now that I am in a wheelchair. Perhaps it's a tendency to be more of a voyeur in life or to participate in different ways.

Many people also reported enjoying spectator sports and, where possible, going to the cinema. A new or continued interest in painting had also been a source of pleasure and of sense of achievement for some individuals. A number also said that they had taken up practical work such as clock and electrical repairs.

Others had taken up academic studies after their injuries. Sometimes this was seen to be a route to employment. However, quite often academic study was pursued simply for the enjoyment and sense of achievement gained. Some individuals were taking part in various Open University courses. Such courses were considered particularly convenient, since the individuals concerned were able to work in their own homes and to spread their studies over a number of years. In this way, they were able to pace their work to suit their own health and time requirements.

A few related how they had become highly involved in helping others through voluntary work and in local community action or political groups:

> I think I feel more satisfied now with my leisure activities than before my accident. My heaviest involvement is with the political side of things—the Labour Party, and that was something I just decided I wanted to get involved with—since then, I've got more heavily involved in the organisation—I'm one of those people who like to get involved in organisation . . . . I think it's very possible I wouldn't [have been involved in this but for the accident] because after I'd finished four 'A' levels I was applying for jobs. I think I would have tried to get a job and then I wouldn't have had the time to get involved in organisations outside.

While such activities and interests had taken a long time to develop, they were clearly a particularly positive aspect of people's lives after they returned home.

For a few individuals, leisure activities did not involve other people to any significant extent. For the majority, however, opportunities for social contact were seen as an integral part of leisure activity itself. Therefore, we shall now broaden out the discussion to consider how people felt about their social lives and the kinds of problems they had experienced.

SOCIAL LIFE

Over 80% of the people we interviewed either were satisfied or expressed only minor dissatisfaction with their social contacts (Table 5.1). As with leisure activities, a lower percentage of paraplegics, as opposed to tetraplegics, expressed marked or severe dissatisfaction with the extent of their social contacts (see Creek *et al.*, 1987:151). There would seem to be a number of possible reasons for this, which we have already started to outline. First, there is the issue of mobility: people with lower-level lesions often found it easier to get out and about than those with higher lesions. Second, there is the differential employment opportunities for people with different levels of lesion (see Chapter 8). There is also the issue of the kinds of leisure activities that people were able to pursue: some activities afforded greater opportunities for social contact than did others—for example, sporting activities. On the other hand, people with complete tetraplegia were more likely to be living with other people and, therefore, have regular social contact in a domestic setting. Dependence on other people to go and see friends, however, also remained a problem for some. Indeed, several people in this situation felt that both their leisure activities and social lives were constrained by the attendance of carers:

> If I go to see my friends I don't want to have to take my Mum with me.

> The whole problem about disability is relying on someone else. It's not the disability, it's the reliance. The problems with disability are—'it's either my freedom or your freedom'—It's about *freedom*, not just for me but for someone else as well.

Those who worked were also more likely to have satisfactory social contacts (see Creek *et al.*, 1987:155). One of the major reasons people had for wishing to get back to work was to join in a normal pattern of social life. Many people commented on the importance of seeing other people in their work. This was often the case, even though work could sometimes mean that people did not have a great deal of time to meet with friends outside working hours. Conversely, people not in employment often emphasised the subsequent lack of social contact:

> You can feel very lonely—then I go out and get a pint . . . . I see a lot less of people than when I was working . . . it's a problem if you let it become so.

Being employed could also often mean having greater financial resources and, therefore, a greater likelihood of being mobile and able to go out and pursue leisure activities and make social contacts.

However, the situation for people who were retired was slightly different. All of the retired individuals in our sample were rated as being satisfied with their social contacts, despite the fact that they often had fewer friends than they had before their accidents. One important reason for this was that many of the older people's social contacts tended to centre around family and neighbours, rather than outside pursuits such as sporting activities.

Despite the highly satisfactory experiences of some individuals, many people felt that there had been a noticeable decline in the level of their social contacts over time once they had returned home from hospital:

> For the first 12 months they were always coming to see me or asking me out and then they dwindled away—they tend to forget . . . it's hard to explain, years ago they used to ask me to go here and there and now they don't—whether they don't want to be bothered with a chap in a wheelchair—I don't know. There are one or two—I suppose they are your true mates aren't they—they stick to you no matter what happens.

> I think relations became increasingly strained between me and my friends because of the nature of their interests and what my interests had been . . . my sort of inability to take part in physical activities increasing, breaking away from that set of friends.

As these comments demonstrate, some people did find that they still had quite a number of friends from before their injury; often people were quite understanding of the fact that relationships might have changed over time, in any case. Nevertheless, a number of individuals felt that they only had a limited number of close friends to whom they were able to talk about problems of a personal or intimate nature:

> 99% of people of my own age would not understand things I have gone through.

This same person also said that he saw more of older people, who:

> ... can understand me better—with my own age I feel more fatherly or older brother. I feel it as a barrier—that's why I can't talk to them—also people don't want to know you when you're down ... I've learnt not to talk about things.

Over time, however, people were usually able to resolve many of these difficulties. Indeed, most said that they did have at least one or two very good friends with whom they could talk about anything, however intimate. Certainly, as the years passed, most people found that their social lives became more satisfying. Nevertheless, a few individuals still felt that they had learned to become very reticent about problems they had experienced since the injury, even with very close friends and family.

Some individuals also spoke about the effect of their presence on others as a limiting factor in their social life. A few people, for example, felt that they were a burden to their friends, holding them back from normal activities and from being able to engage in social activities in a carefree and spontaneous manner. Most people, however, did have a few friends who had stayed with them throughout. A few had developed very close relationships with other spinally injured people while they were in hospital, which they had kept up after they had returned home. They had (as they pointed out) been through a lot together and this, undoubtedly, had often brought them closer together. Others had made good friends with people through disabled sports or other such groups. In fact, several individuals recalled that their relationships with other spinally injured people was a major factor in their rehabilitation while in hospital. On the other hand, some clearly did not wish to make friends only with other disabled people:

> At the moment I can't or maybe I don't want to mix with people that are in wheelchairs all the time—I still want to mix, meet and be with people that are quite normal .... I don't see why if I am in a wheelchair I should be any exception.

A particularly significant aspect of social life for a large number of the people we interviewed concerned personal and sexual relationships. This was also a part of their lives which many individuals found to be most restricted—particularly when they first went home. Consequently, this also tended to be the area in which the highest levels of dissatisfaction were expressed (see Creek *et al.*, 1987:166). This problem was very often exacerbated by the lack of counselling on matters of sexuality at the spinal unit. This subject will be discussed further in Chapter 6.

For those wishing to develop relationships, the most frequently mentioned problem was making the first contact:

> Brief encounters do create enormous problems—it does worry me— everything I've tried so far has failed miserably . . . if you have a longer-term relationship with someone that understands the physical problem is overcome with a psychological one, but on a first encounter basis it's rather different because that in itself leads to a lack of confidence—I can analyse it myself and can quite see it but it's another thing to talk it through with somebody.

> This is where the one night stands don't exist anymore. It takes longer now to introduce yourself to somebody and explain to them what you are about, what your capabilities are and everything else.

As we have seen in relation to other aspects of people's social and leisure activities, the lack of spontaneity associated with the presence of family members and/or carers was often an inhibiting factor:

> It must be difficult for someone to be with me knowing my mother's sat in the front room. The privacy is really gone.

However, a few individuals said that the importance of the family unit to their sense of well-being and security was so great that they could not consider developing intimate relationships. Usually, this kind of comment was made by people with higher-level lesions who felt that their dependence on their families was too great for them to disturb their normal relationship patterns in this way.

Even where difficulties with first encounters were overcome, some younger people still felt that they would be an unattractive prospect for any partner contemplating a long-term relationship or marriage:

> A lot of women aren't interested, are they? No offence, but you're in a wheelchair. People like you to be perfect don't they?. . . People in general, especially women, talk to you more, they don't feel threatened—they don't think you're chatting them up.

A few of these individuals clearly felt that they would consider it unfair to put the burden of a disabled partner on anybody. This was particularly so for those who were more severely disabled where they felt that the burden of care would fall to any prospective partner. A few individuals, for example, felt that it would be unfair for a wife to be a wife and nurse and that such a relationship would be unfulfilling for both partners.

Nevertheless, despite the reservations raised by a few individuals concerning long-term relationships and the problems associated with making first contacts, most people found that their confidence increased significantly over time. Thus, many were eventually able to develop satisfactory relationships, often leading to marriage.

More generally, we have seen that people's satisfaction with their social lives and leisure activities improved with time. However, there were further factors other than time which were also found to be significant. Among these, perhaps the most important concerns independence in mobility and the availability of adequate transport. Therefore, we shall complete this chapter with a discussion of the kinds of restrictions on their mobility which people experienced and, more specifically, the effects of these on their social and leisure activities..

PERSONAL MOBILITY AND WHEELCHAIR USE

Reliable and comfortable wheelchairs are usually fundamental to the personal mobility of people with a spinal cord injury; over 80% of our sample were wheelchair users. However, many people had experienced a wide range of problems with their wheelchairs—particularly standard NHS models. The most common sources of dissatisfaction were poor design, problems of getting efficient servicing and the very high financial costs of both repairs and new wheelchairs (see Creek *et al.*, 1987:174–84).

One specific aspect of wheelchair design which caused problems for many individuals—particularly tetraplegics—was the weight of standard issue NHS models. Several people complained that the heavier models were uncomfortable; even more reported difficulty in pushing themselves. This not only placed practical restrictions on where the wheelchairs could be used, but often also led to reduced incentive to maximise mobility.

These problems with wheelchairs obviously placed restrictions on both the quality of and the opportunities for people's leisure activities. Conversely, the advantages of lightweight, manoeuvrable wheelchairs were also highlighted by several people in the context of both being able to engage in sporting activities and accessibility in the workplace.

Others also mentioned the restrictions on the use of outdoor electric wheelchairs as placing further limitations on their leisure activities.

In fact, the recent Government-commissioned review of the ALAC Service (the *McColl Report*: DHSS, 1986) had also highlighted the widespread nature of these kinds of difficulties which face all wheelchair users—not just those with spinal injuries. The *McColl Report* has recommended that greater attention should be paid to individual requirements and that the criteria for supplying outdoor electric wheelchairs should be widened (DHSS, 1986:8–10). It is hoped that the planned implementation of this recommendation will eventually lead to improvements for wheelchair users and the removal of unnecessary restrictions on their mobility. However, the experience of the people we interviewed suggests that the situation will only be fully resolved when users are able to choose whatever wheelchair is suitable to their self-defined requirements. In this respect, unfortunately, the *McColl Report* does not go far enough.

PRIVATE TRANSPORT

Just as comfortable and reliable wheelchairs are essential to personal mobility, so the use of a car was seen by many people to be a crucially important necessity. Often the use of a car could mean the difference between an independent, active social life and restricted mobility, or even social isolation.

> I knew if I was going to have any sense of mobility, it was going to have to be a car.

> Without the car I'd be lost.

However, the importance of car ownership is not simply restricted to the question of mobility—although this is, of course, fundamental. People also discussed the wider implications—both financial and social—of car ownership for many aspects of daily living. In particular, having a car can make a very significant difference to a person's chances of working after discharge. (For more detailed discussion of the wider implications of private transport, see Creek *et al.*, 1987:184–99.)

THE IMPLICATIONS OF CAR OWNERSHIP FOR SOCIAL AND LEISURE ACTIVITIES

On a practical level, car ownership obviously greatly increases mobility. Thus, many aspects of daily living become that much easier and a desire for an active and independent life-style can become a reality. We have already pointed to some of the implications of personal transport for social and leisure activities. Table 5.2 shows that people who drove their own cars consistently expressed the greatest satisfaction with their social life and leisure activities.

At a day-to-day level, the capacity for independent mobility obviously has a cumulative effect on the quality of life in general. The ability to participate in a wider range of leisure activities increases the potential for making satisfactory social contacts. Where this can be achieved spontaneously, the quality of such social contacts is un-doubtedly enhanced even further. Ultimately, being able to drive can make the difference between wanting independence and actually achieving it:

> If it wasn't for my old boss buying me a car, I don't know what I would have done. Before I had my car it was terrible—you couldn't get out . . . if you wanted something doing you had to ask someone else for it—it was chronic. Now if I get asked, I've got my own car. I can go out and see friends now.

However, for those who did not drive themselves, the reliance on other people to actually drive their cars for them often carried a parallel dilution of independence. Social and leisure activities often had to be arranged around the times when drivers were available. These did not always necessarily coincide with the arrangements people would actually have preferred, given complete freedom of choice. The loss of spontaneity and feelings of being dependent on others for mobility were often a source of considerable frustration:

> I think when I got the car it made a tremendous difference because it gave me an amazing amount of independence—I could go to College on my own and I didn't have to have a lift with my mother and I could go out to other social things on my own—I think it was that that made the real difference.

> I don't like the loss of independence. I would much rather drive because then I am totally independent that way.

In most cases, people who did not have a car said that this was primarily for financial reasons. However, for a few people driving a car was felt to be too much of a problem physically, even with special adaptations. A few individuals also mentioned that they found the process of transferring from wheelchair to car to be an obstacle. This was particularly the case for people with higher-level lesions:

> It would certainly make life better if I could drive myself but you've got

Table 5.2 Relationship between car ownership and satisfaction with leisure activities and social contacts

Level of satisfaction	Car owner/driver		Car owner/non-driver		No car		Row totals	
	Social contacts	Leisure activities	Social contacts	Leisure activities	Social contacts	Leisure activities	Social contacts	Leisure activities
Satisfied (%)	70.0	57.5	23.5	27.8	44.4	33.3	53.3	44.7
Minor dissatisfaction (%)	22.5	32.5	41.2	33.3	33.3	44.4	29.3	35.5
Marked or severe dissatisfaction (%)	7.5	10.0	35.2	38.9	22.2	22.2	17.4	19.7
Base totals	100.0	100.0	100.0	100.0	100.0	100.0	100.0	100.0
	(40)	(40)	(17)	(18)	(18)	(18)	(75)	(76)

this transferring business and I just don't want to do it. It's just too much for me personally. . . my hope is that one day they are going to come up with a car where you just drive straight in and I know they are making moves because I've seen one but the price of it was staggering, £10 000, so I'll wait.

It may well be, therefore, that driving a car is not always a practical way to meet everyone's individual mobility requirements. However, this is not to say that their requirements could not be met by alternative means. The provision of cars capable of taking a wheelchair via an electric 'arm' or lift would mitigate the problem of transferring. In other cases the regular availability of drivers at times to suit people's needs may be a solution.

PUBLIC TRANSPORT

Public transport was not a highly significant aspect of mobility for the people we interviewed: over 80% never used the bus at all and over 90% never used trains (Creek *et al.*, 1987:200). This reflects the fact that most public transport provision fails to accommodate the needs of people with physical impairments. In view of this situation, the previous comments on the importance of private transport for mobility become even more urgent.

Even for the few individuals who were regular bus or train users, public transport was not without its problems. Once again, in order to use these services, people were still very much dependent on having helpers available to lift them on and off the train or bus. Furthermore, some parts of the public transport system—particularly underground tube trains—remain almost totally inaccessible, even if helpers are available.

People who did not have any private transport tended to make more use of public transport services. However, even among this group, overall usage was very low and mostly restricted to occasional use only. Obviously, it is plausible to suggest that people without cars were likely to have less choice about having to use public transport, whatever obstacles they may have to overcome. This is even more likely when we consider the problems of friends and relations with cars not always being available at the required times.

CONCLUSIONS

As we have seen in this chapter, the interpersonal relationships and social and leisure activities which people develop are a crucial aspect of the disability career following their return to the community. While there were wide variations in how different individuals developed new activities and areas of interest, there were also certain common features in their experiences which should be highlighted.

First, the large majority of people we interviewed felt that these areas of their lives had improved over time. Usually this was a gradual process, sometimes involving changing expectations and the development of different areas of interest from those people had before their injuries. Second, both opportunities for, and satisfaction with, leisure and social activities were closely interlinked: engaging in leisure activities—particularly outside the home—provided many people with important social contacts as well as the opportunity to develop either old or new interests. Third, the way in which people actually perceived their opportunities for leisure and social activities was found to be more important than any actual restrictions in determining levels of satisfaction.

Nevertheless, there were various restrictions on leisure and social activities which people had to face. For some, the necessity of having to rely on others—particularly for transport—meant that spontaneity and freedom of choice were restricted. People who were not working or in education often found that they had too much leisure time, without enough meaningful activity to fill it. An important factor in this was often the problem of lack of finance, which, in turn, could also reduce an individual's chances of obtaining adequate personal transport.

One particularly important aspect of social life mentioned by many people concerned the development of personal and sexual relationships. This was an area of people's lives which many found took the longest to develop satisfactorily. As with social and leisure activities generally, the presence of others—usually family members or other carers—was often an inhibiting factor. This was particularly the case for people with higher-level lesions, some of whom felt that their dependence on their families was too great to jeopardise by the development of new personal relationships. This is obviously a sensitive issue which, once again, raises a question mark over the blanket assumption that discharge back to the family is the best strategy for all people with higher-level lesions.

Finally, we examined the effects of restrictions on personal mobility which people often experienced. Regarding wheelchair use and personal mobility, there were wide-ranging complaints about both the design and the supply of wheelchairs. Many of these were seen as easily avoidable if only greater consideration could be given to individual requirements. It is hoped that the implementation of the McColl recommendations regarding the ALAC Service will lead to improvements in the future.

Throughout this chapter, we have stressed the importance of

personal transport and car ownership. For many people, being independently mobile was the most important factor in being able to enjoy satisfying social and leisure activities. For people who either did not own a car or were dependent on others to drive them, there were problems with drivers not being available at the time preferred and, once again, the lack of spontaneity, which placed restrictions on the enjoyment of social and leisure activities. Often this situation was exacerbated by the inaccessibility of the public transport system, which meant that most people hardly ever used buses, tubes or trains.

Clearly, mobility is of crucial importance to people with a spinal injury, in both their social and their working lives. It is essential, therefore, that the kinds of restrictions on mobility which are often faced should be reduced as far as possible. As we have seen, when these restrictions are removed, people are able to develop satisfactory social lives and meaningful leisure activities.

CHAPTER 6

Perceptions of Medical and Social Services

INTRODUCTION

In this chapter, we attempt to convey spinal-cord-injured individuals' perceptions of health and social services both during the hospitalisation period and in the community, following discharge. Professionals play a key role in determining access to, and delivery of, a whole range of services both in hospital and in the community. Thus, they can have a significant effect on the direction of the disability career.

Government policies and professional interventions regarding people with disabilities are increasingly geared towards providing effective care in the community (CCETSW, 1974; Barclay Committee, 1982; ACC, 1985; Audit Commission, 1986). It is important, therefore, to consider how present service provision is experienced and evaluated by the people who actually use the services available. More specifically, in the context of this study, it is necessary to examine whether or not these services meet the self-defined needs of people with spinal cord injury.

A recent report (Audit Commission, 1986) points to an urgent need for wide-ranging organisational changes and new approaches from service providers if effective community care is to become a reality. From the perspective of disabled people who use health and community services, there are three key issues: choice, control and adequacy. The questions of choice and adequacy revolve around whether or not the range of services available is wide enough and sufficiently flexible to meet people's individual needs. Closely related to this is the question of whether needs themselves are defined primarily by the users, or by the providers, of services. In other words, whether or not disabled people have sufficient control over the type and level of services provided.

A further critical feature of current service provision highlighted in the Audit Commission report concerns the lack of co-ordination between the multiple agencies involved. Findings from other research on the use of community services have also pointed to the fragmentary nature of service delivery and organisation as an important factor in the failure to provide adequate support to disabled people and their families (Blaxter, 1980; Glendinning, 1986; Owens, 1987).

The pressing need for co-ordination and follow-up, particularly once an individual has returned to the community, is also a major theme to emerge from the analysis of service provision in the present study. What services are actually received and whether they are adequate for people's needs is often due to quite arbitrary factors: where an individual lives, who he knows, what he knows, or simply the attitude of the service personnel he happens to be dealing with.

Our study did not specifically set out to examine the way in which hospital and community services are organised. Nevertheless, the experiences of the people we interviewed highlight the fact that there are some significant gaps between what spinal-cord-injured people feel they need and what services are willing or able to provide. These gaps in provision need to be examined within a critical framework which will allow us to highlight the areas where the need for improvement or change is most urgent. Consequently, when examining spinal-cord-injured people's perceptions of particular services, we shall also focus on the wider issues of choice, control, co-ordination and adequacy which emerged as underlying many of the problems experienced.

The questions of choice and flexibility in the meeting of individual needs are particularly relevant to the provision of services for people with spinal cord injury. First, as we have seen in Chapter 4, there is genuine diversity in how each individual subjectively experiences spinal cord injury as a 'significant life event'. Likewise, each will be placed in a different set of social and material circumstances. Furthermore, both the subjects's subjective and his objective situations will change over time. Consequently, what he requires of medical and social services will not remain static. Yet many of the personnel involved in the 'rehabilitation' process appear to have a fairly inflexible approach as to how their particular service should be delivered. All too often this fails to match up to what the people who use these services expect or desire. This situation leads both to some critical gaps in service provision and to the wrong kind of service being provided at the wrong time.

Furthermore, as far as service provision is concerned, 'rehabilitation' often appears to end at the time of discharge. People tend to be left to cope without support—just at the time when a whole new range of emotional, social and practical problems are starting to become apparent. The consequences of the lack of follow-up by the community services will be illustrated in subsequent parts of this chapter. The general trend is also highlighted by the quantitative summary of levels of contact with various professionals—particularly social workers and occupational therapists—shown in Table 6.1. (For more detailed statistics, see Creek *et al.*, 1987, Chapter 9.)

Table 6.1 Levels of contact with medical and social services

Contact with	In hospital	On discharge	At interview
Social worker (%)	81.6	53.9	31.2
Occupational therapist (%)	–	32.9	19.5
District nurse (%)	–	47.4	41.6
GP (%)	–	78.9	84.4
Domiciliary physiotherapist (%)	–	15.8	15.8
Home help (%)	–	–	10.4
Other professionals (%)	–	–	25.0

Base total = 77.
– = data not collected.

Finally, it seems clear that any restrictions on choice, control and adequacy which are experienced are closely linked to the way services are organised and delivered by the professionals (and their employers) who provide them. From the consumers' perspective, a critical feature of this situation is that the professionals who control access to the services they need often effectively define their needs for them. Furthermore, without adequate information, consumers face great difficulties in gaining any measure of control over how their needs should be met, or even whether they will be met at all (Blaxter, 1980; Wilding, 1982; Oliver, 1983; BCODP, 1987).

COUNSELLING AND FAMILY SUPPORT

The implications of professional control over access to services are wide-ranging. On entry to hospital, for example, people are immediately dependent on medical professionals providing the information necessary for them to understand their changed circumstances and the physical consequences of their injuries. As we have seen in Chapter 3, however, this vital information is often either withheld or inappropriately handled. The question of how individuals with a spinal cord injury should be informed about their injuries leads on to a wider discussion of the kind of emotional and practical support required during the hospitalisation period. Our data reveal a significant lack of support—particularly in the area of counselling—for both the individuals who are spinal-cord-injured and their families. Within the hospital services, including those at the spinal unit, there is a strong emphasis on the medical and physical aspects of rehabilitation. The majority of people in our study reported the medical care they received within the spinal unit to be of a very high quality. However, the very efficiency with which such medical care is delivered often seems to create an atmosphere of impersonality and regimentation which many individuals experienced as unsupportive of their more intimate and critical needs.

One of the most frequently mentioned areas of unmet need concerned counselling over fertility and sexuality:

> I came out of there as blank as a dodo—there was never any direct conversation with any of the doctors about fertility—only what you picked up on the ward—no one ever explained that side of it to me—whether I can have kids or anything.

> There was some counselling in the broadest sense but it wasn't really dealt with on an individual basis—again it was a period of instability in the sense you don't really quite know where you were going.

The lack of counselling over fertility and sexuality during the hospitalisation period also has longer-term effects since, once they leave the spinal unit, people find that there are very few places in the community where they can go for further advice and support. While anxiety about sexuality and sexual relations sometimes arose in hospital, several individuals we interviewed perceived a need for longer-term support after discharge, since it is often only when they leave the unit that any problems are actually manifested:

> I'm not sure it would have been of so much value then [in the spinal unit] as later—I would have welcomed a contact point to be able to go back for advice when I really needed help much later—whether it should be done locally or at Stoke Mandeville, I don't know.

Some people also mentioned that they would have appreciated advice following discharge, because they were contemplating long-term relationships, or marriage. Several also expressed great resentment that there had been no sperm testing or routine banking—which is the norm in some other spinal units. For many people, the chances of saving sperm are fairly low, but this was rarely explained. Again, the realisation that they may not be able to father children is a potential source of stress and anxiety for many spinal-cord-injured men and their partners. Clearly, more could be done in the way of providing information and support.

These kinds of problems also illustrate that it is not only the individual with a spinal cord injury who needs support and advice; often there is an equally urgent need for family support, from both the hospital and the community services. Within the hospital services, not only is there a strong emphasis on the medical and physical aspects of rehabilitation, but also this activity is obviously focused on 'the patient'. This tends to make the hospital environment particularly unsupportive for relatives in terms of both their practical and emotional needs:

There should really be somebody who could talk to you and help you to face up to it. I was given a book *So Now You're Paralysed* and reading that is pretty dreadful really—all by yourself, just reading that and facing all the gruesome facts. I think I must have been encouraged—someone must have told me to go and buy it—no one actually followed that up, I mean, you went off to your sort of sterile room that Stoke Mandeville allowed you to have for a bit. It's very kind. They give you a sterile, clean hospital visitors' room and you sit on a sterile bed and you think, 'What on earth has happened?' You really do need somebody at that point I think.

The tendency for the needs of family members to be overlooked is partly related to the overstretched resources of the spinal unit. However, this was sometimes due to the practice of excluding family members from decisions about the care of their relatives. For example, several relatives who participated in the interviews expressed their resentment at having to leave the wards during turning and other medical tasks. Not surprisingly, since they would usually be the ones to provide care support following discharge, the relatives felt that they should be more closely involved from the start.

What advice relatives were given also tended to be restricted to purely functional aspects of caring—for example, how to perform a manual evacuation, turning, lifting and dressing—without consideration of how they might feel about this. There was often very little opportunity to discuss how the need to provide long-term care would affect relatives' own lives and their interpersonal relationships.

It is fairly clear, therefore, that lack of counselling—for both the individual with a spinal injury and his family—represents a significant gap in service provision during the hospitalisation period. The need for counselling and emotional support as defined by spinal-cord-injured people themselves does not seem to match particularly well with the hospital services approach to rehabilitation, which is primarily focused on the medical and physical, rather than the personal and social, aspects of spinal cord injury:

I think this whole counselling thing, at that point [being told about the nature of the injury] and at other points when there are terrific things to work out—looking back now, I think there was a huge lack.

Physically, I was weak. Looking back, I can't remember half of it—just the shock—and you are all full of drugs, and at that time it didn't make much difference [the lack of counselling] because at the time you were so preoccupied, you didn't even bother thinking about it.

I think there is a need for some sort of psychological guidance or treatment, psychological discussion or something. The trouble was, all they did then was they called in a psychiatrist.

Clearly, even if people were not sure exactly what form of counselling they required, it was not 'psychiatric' treatment. The need for counselling does not stem from any psychological disorder, but rather from the anxieties and uncertainties about the interruption to normality which spinal cord injury undoubtedly creates in the acute post-injury period. Furthermore, the lack of counselling may itself have the effect of increasing such anxieties.

There is also a critical gap between needs and services in the apparent failure to integrate the needs of family members and to provide any follow-up support when it is most needed following discharge. Several people recalled that the hospitalisation period is not the appropriate time to make long-term decisions, as they were often not well enough, physically, to make considered assessments of their situation. More importantly, however, the hospital environment does not provide any indication of what living in the community will be like. Consequently, it is in the post-discharge period that the greatest need will arise:

> There is no way within the hospital environment that it's going to prepare you for what you are going to face when you get out.

> They really need someone who can come round—a visiting counsellor—about 6 months after to talk to you. The strains come after about 6 months—the cracks start showing.

HOSPITAL SOCIAL WORK SERVICE

Overall, nearly 82% of the people we interviewed had some contact with a medical social worker while in hospital. There were, however, wide variations in the level and quality of support received. First, people who were most recently injured (within the previous 4 years) were significantly more likely to have been in contact with a social worker than in earlier years. Furthermore, while individual social workers were often very supportive, inadequate staffing levels and lack of time constrained the service into a limited 'problem solving' role. Consequently, while social workers were able to deal with specific housing and welfare needs as they arose, they were often unable to provide the wider support and advice which people wanted. This inevitably led to gaps in the information and advice received—particularly regarding where and how to obtain other social services following discharge:

> There was no social worker for much of the time you were there—I was given a bundle of leaflets about financial benefits but not much else. I got more advice from another patient's family.

All the social worker wanted to know was—'Haven't you seen your family?' so that was that. They work on the easiest thing for them. They just try to palm you off the easiest way to get you down as finished, out of the way.

It must be difficult for them to know how to approach people—they've only got such a short time to get to know people, but she got on with it, got all the paper work done.

The lack of adequate information felt by many people we interviewed also illustrates the consequences of the inflexible professional control over access to services discussed in the introduction to this chapter. Several people felt that they were in a 'catch-22' situation regarding social work advice. Without adequate information about the full range of social services available to them, they are not always able to exercise any choice over the service they receive:

The social worker was very good, but she was very restricted because she was the only one. She did sort out a lot of things for me, but you need so much more. You need explaining, and she needed time and you don't know the questions to ask or where to go for services.

You have to know what to ask for and you have to ask for everything.

For the social workers themselves, the constraints on their own resources mean that they are often only able to respond to the most pressing claims on their time. Consequently, people sometimes felt that the onus was on them to work out their own requirements. This was particularly the case over decisions about living and occupational arrangements following discharge:

My pushing and seeking out people made it work for me—the alternative was that they kicked you out into a home or else they kicked you out to your parents. If you hadn't got a family they discharged you to your general hospital, that happened—if you wanted anything else and didn't fit the pattern . . . . I spent a long time in Stoke waiting . . . you must be persistent, don't settle for things that are wrong or that you are unhappy with.

These kinds of problems with the social work service are compounded by a lack of follow-up and co-ordination with services outside the hospital. Several people reported that arrangements hospital social workers had made on their behalf were not followed by the community services once they had left the unit. This situation largely results from wider administrative requirements of social service provision which are beyond the control of social workers at the spinal unit; following discharge, responsibility for social work support reverts to the local social service department. The combination of the distances involved and the change of administrative jurisdiction undoubtedly makes it very difficult for social workers at the spinal unit to ensure that arrangements they have made for housing, adaptations, home helps, etc., are actually carried out. Some of the longer-term consequences of such lack of co-ordination and follow-up will be discussed later in the chapter.

PHYSIOTHERAPY AND OCCUPATIONAL THERAPY

In contrast to many of the other hospital and community services used by people in our study, physiotherapy at the spinal unit was regularly reported in particularly positive terms. It is, perhaps, also significant that it was the only service which people did not feel was under-resourced. Many people not only found the physiotherapy staff to be very supportive, but also appreciated their approach to rehabilitation and found it to be of great practical benefit—particularly when they had actually left the unit:

> They were super—I couldn't wish for better. They've got the right attitude—getting on with it rather than letting you lie there thinking it's the end. They seemed bloody hard at the time—then you realised they were doing you a lot of good.

> The physiotherapy staff were very good—it's not so much learning, it's telling you—this is what's left of your body, make the most of it—I really got on well with them.

Nevertheless, there were some people who still considered the unit's approach to rehabilitation to be too regimented and not responsive enough to individual preferences:

> I always felt Stoke Mandeville's rehabilitation was a bit—like a conveyor belt thing—you were put on it and to some extent you didn't have much say.

> You didn't have any say in your treatment—if you didn't like it—tough luck—it was standard procedure to do certain things.

These qualifications to the generally positive assessment made of the service highlight the related questions of choice and of patients having an input in decisions regarding their rehabilitation. While some individuals were critical, they did not deny either the value of physiotherapy or the efficiency with which the service was delivered. The important point was that their own assessment of where physiotherapy ranked in relation to their other priorities did not always match that of the physiotherapist.

Consequently, many people felt that they would have preferred a greater say in when and how they used the physiotherapy service. The service was most efficiently utilised, therefore, when individuals' own preferences were taken into account. Indeed, this is how some physiotherapists were seen to have approached their work—as a partnership. Significantly, the most positive response of all came from an individual who had had exactly this sort of partnership while at the unit:

> I have nothing but praise for them—they are the backbone of the place. I was a difficult patient—I knew what I wanted to do and I was going to do it my way. Rather than try to make me do what she wanted, she'd make me do what I wanted the way she wanted me to do it—so far as I'm concerned, she did it absolutely right—she and I worked together to solve my problems.

In contrast to physiotherapy, perceptions of the occupational therapy service were almost universally negative:

> The standard overall I thought was very poor—we had the workshop, but the expectations of OT were too low and there wasn't enough scope for someone to really pursue something that really interested them—the occupational therapists could do a lot more than they do—but it's got this middle-aged married woman earning a few bob part-time image—and until it's given professional respect it will never increase its potential.

> I didn't think much of the OT—it was flower arranging, passing time—which didn't appeal to me much. OT is a bit limited because it's so small [they] need a bigger unit, more staff and a bigger variety of skills.

Lack of resources and the very limited scope of the activities undertaken meant quite simply that most people considered that they derived little or no practical benefit from the service. Once again, several people also felt that they did not have the opportunity to set their own priorities regarding the type of activities they were engaged in. Consequently, they were often simply disinterested. Clearly, greater choice and responsiveness to individual preferences would go some way to improving the adequacy of the occupational therapy service.

GENERAL PRACTITIONER SERVICE

It might be expected that the local GP would be the key figure in the ongoing process of rehabilitation once people had left the spinal unit. For the majority, however, this was not the case. As with the receiving hospitals, the level of specialist knowledge about spinal cord injury among GPs was generally low. Very often people found that, when they were dealing with GPs, roles were reversed—with 'the patients' being the expert on spinal cord injury:

> Once I left there [the spinal unit] I was back in the hands of people who knew very little about spinal injuries.

> My GP told us he knows nothing about people like us.

> I know far more about my injury—I have absolutely no confidence in my GP.

As a result of the lack of knowledge about spinal cord injury on the part of GPs, some people felt that they had received inappropriate or unnecessary treatment:

> We only called him out once, he came and went all panicky and sent me off to hospital for tests—they didn't find anything wrong—I think he just overreacted.

There were also instances reported where GPs' actions had caused practical inconvenience over financial and welfare matters, or, as in the following example, had led to problems related to employment:

> The GP is totally useless—she signed me off for work before I was able to after pressure sores.

As these examples illustrate, people were often unable to get appropriate service even over fairly routine matters. As with any other patient group, people with a spinal cord injury expect to receive appropriate medical advice and treatment when medical complications arise. However, lack of familiarity on the part of GPs seems to make this unnecessarily difficult.

Although apparently in the minority, there were some GPs who were prepared to acknowledge their limitations and took the time to learn from spinal-cord-injured individuals about their needs. However, many people we interviewed found not only that their GPs were lacking in knowledge about their medical condition, but also that they were not prepared to learn or take an interest. Thus, people were sometimes effectively denied access to the services they needed. Some were prepared to return to the spinal unit whenever they had a medical problem, assuming that the spinal unit was prepared to take them. A few had their need for routine medical care met by, for example, a particularly accommodating district nurse. Often, however, people were simply left to cope on their own or with the assistance of their family members:

I don't have any confidence in my GP, I always go to Stoke.

I only saw my GP once on discharge—I was getting very stiff, he just said—'I can't do anything for you, I'm afraid, I don't know anything about your situation, go back to Stoke—ask the experts'. I've had no contact since, he didn't want to know, he'd lost interest in me—he made me feel as if he didn't have time for me.

DISTRICT NURSING SERVICE

Just over 40% of the people in our study were in contact with a district nurse at the time of interview. However, people who had received their injuries most recently were far more likely to have been in contact with the service—particularly immediately following discharge. Conversely, many people injured in earlier years who did not see a district nurse on discharge were still not receiving the service at the time of interview (Creek *et al.*, 1987:295–96).

These differences in levels of contact are indicative of the lack of follow-up and co-ordination characteristic of many of the services used by people with spinal cord injury. Several of the people injured in earlier years have simply never been picked up—either by the local health authority or by their GPs—and have not, therefore, been contacted to find out whether they require the services of a district nurse. Many reported that they were not even aware that the service was available to them. In some cases, there also seemed to be an expectation that family members would be able to cope without assistance:

The district nurse only supplied the bed—she's never been once to see if my wife can cope—my wife has to help me out of the bath and she has to wipe me down. The district nurse is non-existent in this area.

Regarding the quality of service received, people had experienced a great deal of local variation. Different local authorities had quite contrasting policies regarding both the level and type of district nursing service provided. In some cases, the restrictions on personnel resources were compounded by district nurses having to give priority to the needs of other client groups—particularly the elderly. Consequently, the service many people received was felt to be inadequate. The most common sources of dissatisfaction concerned the inflexibility of the service, which very often could not be provided at the times when it was actually most needed:

The district nurse service is getting better—now they come in every day. But there is still a problem with the hours they are available—the earliest they can come in the morning is 8.30, which is rather too late for work, but it's OK because my working hours are flexible. Then, at night, they come much too early—so I don't use them then.

I wish they did come in earlier so that my dad didn't have to help me on the toilet.

Apart from the inflexibility over the times the service is available, these comments also highlight other related problems which were commonly experienced. First, there is the important question of choice: while the quality of nursing care actually received was of a generally high quality, people were not able to influence the time district nurses could visit. Their daily activities, therefore, have to be structured around the service providers' schedule, not their own. Clearly, this can be a source of great inconvenience—particularly for people who are in employment. Many simply did not use the service, for this reason. Similarly, the lack of choice regarding when to be helped in and out of bed was another source of frustration which could be overcome through closer attention to individual needs and preferences.

Nevertheless, some people reported that their district nurse was prepared to give broader support beyond the strict definition of her nursing role. However, the likelihood of obtaining satisfactory service is due to quite arbitrary factors; much depends on the available resources, the policy of particular local health authorities and the disposition of particular nursing personnel.

SOCIAL SERVICES AND SOCIAL WORK SUPPORT

Following discharge, most people's perceived needs focus increasingly upon the area of social, emotional and practical support. Furthermore, such support is seen to be required on an ongoing basis. However, the experiences of the people we interviewed suggest that it is in the area of social services that provision is most lacking. Once again, while some individual social service personnel were extremely supportive of the injured people and their families, the broader pattern of provision reveals a variety of significant inadequacies.

One particularly common problem concerned the long delays many people experienced in getting the personal aids and housing adaptations they needed. Many people, for example, had experienced delays in obtaining housing adaptations which were often caused by lack of liaison between local authority social service and housing departments (see Chapter 7 for further discussion). Such delays were sometimes further exacerbated by the lack of contact with a social worker to follow up and co-ordinate the initial request for adaptations:

> We approached social services about rebuilding the bathroom and kitchen to make it accessible from the wheelchair. It was 2½ to 3 years before anything got done and they weren't at all helpful. They refused to give a penny and said we'd have to do it, but they would help with a ramp— which was already done, and they were only going to pay for half of that.

Personal aids were also a problem:

> When we asked for help with installing a telephone—they wouldn't help or nothing—no way.

> I had a problem getting a special cushion for the wheelchair from the OT— it took 3 months to get the right cushion.

These delays in obtaining services are indicative of the general lack of follow-up among the social services after discharge from hospital. A quantitative indicator of this lack of follow-up is given by the significant decrease in the level of contact which people had with community social workers and occupational therapists between the time of discharge and the time of interview (see Table 6.1).

Obviously, some reduction in the level of contact with social workers and occupational therapists will be expected over time; once necessary aids and adaptations have been provided and other services arranged, the need for follow-up may not be so frequent—although, for some, it will continue over months or years. However, the significant reduction in the level of service provision suggests that this cannot fully explain the lack of follow-up which the people we interviewed experienced.

Even though the need for support and advice may decline in the longer term, such need is in fact greatest in the immediate post-discharge period. Yet only just over half of our sample were in contact with a social worker on discharge, compared with over 80% during the hospitalisation period. The consequences of this lack of follow-up can be further illustrated by some of the extracts from the interviews:

> The social worker came twice—but I would have liked much more advice—I could have done with a great deal more help after discharge. Every time my wife speaks to Stoke about it—they are highly disgusted.

> Nobody wants to do nothing—we never see the social worker—she came the first weekend dad came home, that was all we saw of her.

These reported experiences highlight the breakdown in service provision at the time of discharge, precisely when it is most needed; while hospital social workers and others at the spinal unit had made arrangements with people's local social services, often these were simply not followed up.

The problem of lack of follow-up is compounded by the administrative fragmentation of the various social and other community services. The experiences reported here—and their practical consequences—are similar to those found in previous studies of the use of social services by disabled people and their families (Bradshaw *et al.*, 1977; Blaxter, 1980). These and other studies have suggested that there is an urgent need for a single professional to co-ordinate and advise on the fragmentary services which disabled people need to use (Fox, 1974), although the effectiveness of this has yet to be clearly demonstrated (Glendinning, 1986).

A large number of people we interviewed also felt that there is a need for a regular contact or 'key person' to both advise on and co-ordinate their various requests for services and, most importantly, follow them up with the authorities or departments responsible for their provision:

> I would like to have had a social worker—not so much to advise on personal or family problems—I can do that myself—but to advise me on benefits. I feel I'm getting ripped off on a lot of money I'm entitled to and not getting—but then because I'm lazy, I can't be bothered to go after them—I wouldn't know where to start myself.

> I think it's important to have one key person in the community to co-ordinate all the services. It's confusing with all the different people coming in—no one seems to take responsibility.

A small number of people had received this kind of on-going support, either from a social worker or, in some cases, an occupational therapist. Thus, they were able to obtain the services they required and were far more satisfied with the level of provision than were the large majority of people we interviewed:

> The social worker was very good—she came and just talked—she was really good. She also got us the money for a deposit on a car.

> If we don't know anything we usually phone [the occupational therapist] and she puts us in touch—she's our link. She tells us who can help, but often she does it herself—she got the bed and commode, sorted our extension and finance, we wouldn't have got where we are now if it hadn't been for her. She contacted us 2 months after the accident and organised everything—I think that's why things moved so quickly.

Clearly, there is a need for greater co-ordination of the range of community services available so that consumers can have a real choice in how their needs are met. It has been suggested that social services departments—and occupational therapists in particular—are best placed to take responsibility for such co-ordination. However, most of the evidence also suggests that they are failing to do so (CCETSW, 1974; DHSS, 1978; Howe, 1980; Borsay, 1983).

In the present study, people who were in contact with an occupational therapist reported wide variation in the quality of service received. A few community occupational therapists were able to offer a high degree of generalised and on-going support. Most people, however, did not perceive the service to be either appropriate or adequate to their needs. As with many other services, problems reported included a lack of knowledge about spinal injury, long delays in dealing with requests for services or equipment, and insensitive and unaccommodating professional attitudes.

The likelihood of receiving satisfactory support from the social services, therefore, often depends on the disposition of particular personnel. However, the availability of resources and, most importantly, the policies of the local authorities concerned are also highly relevant factors. Although apparently a minority, some local authorities were sensitive to the needs of people with physical impairments and were committed to policies which were enabling to people living in the community. Furthermore, some people reported that their local social services were prepared to acknowledge the existence of gaps in provision and to attempt to raise the level of support:

> The social services here have been very good—I've been impressed by everything they've done—they seem to be committed to a policy of independent living—they are arranging to find a permanent paid carer to live in. They also found alternative accommodation for me while they were doing the adaptation.

Nevertheless, despite improvements in some areas, many local authorities remained unsupportive. Some people acknowledged that lack of resources were preventing their social service department from providing the level of support required. Some also considered that the level of service provision in their areas had actually declined; again, they usually attributed this to cuts in resources. Nevertheless, understanding the reasons for the low levels of service provision did not make people any less dissatisfied with the lack of support:

> I think they felt so strained in their resources—they couldn't promise anything.

> Until now it hasn't been too much of a problem because I was away at College so it was only holidays, but when I came home for good last September—my mother had 5 months without any help at all.

Often the situation was made worse by the unaccommodating attitude of service personnel with whom people had had contact:

> I wish I'd never met her [social worker], she didn't do a thing for me. She kept trying to tell me what to do—not advising, just telling me where to

go, what to do. She didn't ask for my opinion, she thought—because your legs have gone, your brain has gone with it—she'd decide everything for me.

In addition to the problems of lack of resources and unaccommodating professional attitudes, some people also came up against organisational obstacles to getting the kind of support they needed. In some cases, as in the following example, these problems had actually prevented or delayed people wishing to return home from hospital.

The community service volunteers wanted someone to liaise with in the social services department who could keep an eye on the CSV—they [social services department] just *didn't* want to know—they said they would find another helper—my son was still in Stoke Mandeville Hospital and couldn't come home because I hadn't got anyone – and the day he was due to come home they said they couldn't find anyone so I was left high and dry in the disabled unit. The consultants brought him into the disabled unit until we found someone, so by that time I was beginning to get a bit upset and in the end I rang our MP because it made me *so* cross— he had spent 8 months in hospital and this was standing in the way of [my son] coming home—they [social services department] didn't want to get involved with community service volunteers. So then the MP got on to the head of social services department and it trickled down through and in the end we got a CSV, and that's how it had to be done.

This example also illustrates the lengths people sometimes had to go to in order to obtain the co-operation of the community services. It also raises the 'political' question of what the appropriate relationship between statutory and voluntary agencies in the provision of support services should be. While a detailed discussion of this issue would not be appropriate here, it is useful to consider people's experiences with voluntary agencies and whether or not they were useful in meeting their needs.

THE ROLE OF VOLUNTARY SERVICES

A small number of the people we interviewed had made use of care attendant schemes run by voluntary organisations such as Crossroads and Community Service Volunteers (CSVs). It is useful, therefore, to briefly discuss their perceptions of voluntary schemes and their relation to existing statutory services.

People who had used voluntary care attendant schemes usually compared them very favourably with the services available from statutory agencies. The greatest advantage of the schemes is that they are flexible and responsive to particular individual needs. For example, while some people had had individual care attendants whom they did not find satisfactory, they were often able to arrange replacements with the agencies concerned.

The flexibility of the voluntary schemes is in distinct contrast to most of the reported experiences regarding statutory services. It is interesting to note that some local authority social services departments were prepared to acknowledge that voluntary agencies were filling critical gaps in existing service provision. There also appears to be an increasing recognition in some social service departments that the availability of long-term care support tailored to individual needs is enabling to people who wish to live independently in the community. Consequently, a few individuals found that their local authorities were prepared to liaise with voluntary agencies to assist in the provision of such support:

> I think the attitude has changed now because they [social services] have suddenly realised there is a gap.

> They [social services] appear to be committed to a policy of independent living—they are arranging to find a permanent paid carer to live in.

Unfortunately, however, many local authorities were not as supportive. We have already seen, for example, that some social service departments were actually quite obstructive:

> They [social services] didn't have anyone to help—and yet when we were willing to get a CSV they didn't want to help. It wasn't going to cost them a penny—no money at all—we only wanted a supervisor. Even the social worker—who was excellent—didn't want a CSV.

The previous extract from the interview data also illustrates a further problem some people had experienced when trying to arrange care support outside of existing statutory services. The problem essentially concerns the inability of local authority social service departments to provide cash payments which would allow people to have a completely free hand in the type of care support they obtained:

> At the moment, I have three people whom I nominally call 'social services aides', but I actually recruited myself—trained in my own needs—and whom I relate to on a day-to-day basis. I arranged the times they come in and agreed the hours that they work. All that practically happens is that the social services handles the administration—the local authority pays, but in every other respect the relationship is, as I see it, between them [the aides] and myself and I foster a situation in which they relate to me in that way—as the employer. I am trying to negotiate with the local authority at the moment, to actually formalise the situation but the difficulty is the

legal constraints—the local authority can provide services—but they can't provide cash.

A few individuals, therefore, were able to deal with the inadequacies in existing statutory services by recruiting their own care attendants. In this way, they were able to obtain care support which was more precisely suited to their particular needs and requirements. However, while such arrangements were found to be far more suitable than using statutory services, the need for administrative liaison with local authority departments still made the process unnecessarily complex. Their experience suggests that—assuming suitable services are available—straightforward cash support from local authority sources would be particularly advantageous. This would, perhaps, allow for greater flexibility and complete freedom of choice, thus enabling people to obtain the kind of care support most suited to their requirements.

CONCLUSIONS

The major theme of this chapter has been the lack of co-ordination and follow-up of service provision—particularly when people return to the community. Administrative fragmentation of the various services provided often fails to match the self-defined needs of people with spinal cord injury themselves. Consequently, many people experienced critical gaps in the level of support they had received. Everyone we interviewed had their own individual perceptions of what they required from the various services available. Such needs did not remain static; the kind of support required over the disability career is characterised by changing combinations of medical, emotional, practical and social support. However, administrative fragmentation and service providers' narrow definitions of need often mean that services are too inflexible to respond to people's evolving requirements.

Hospital services were primarily focused on the medical and physical aspects of rehabilitation. But many people perceived a critical gap in the provision of emotional support and counselling. Following discharge, concern was focused increasingly on practical and social support. For the majority, however, return to the community marked a distinct discontinuity in the level and quality of support received—particularly from the social services.

Many people felt that they were being left to cope with minimal support. Common problems concerned long delays in obtaining particular services; unaccommodating professional attitudes; and poor liaison between different statutory agencies and between statutory and voluntary agencies. Many also felt that service providers should pay closer attention to individual choices over when and how services should be delivered. A small number of individuals had attempted— with varying degrees of success—to obtain care support outside of existing statutory services. While these arrangements were found to be more suitable to individual requirements than were statutory services, the individuals concerned still faced problems due to poor liaison with local social service departments.

Despite some improvements in certain services in recent years, the overall level and quality of service provision was not found to be adequate to meet the needs of people with spinal cord injury and their families. The experiences reported here clearly indicate a need for considerable improvements: increased resources, greater co-ordination and responsiveness to individuals' own definitions of need would seem to be the most urgent improvements required.

CHAPTER 7

Housing and Accommodation

INTRODUCTION

Finding suitable accommodation or adapting existing accommodation can be a major problem for someone who has to resume his life in a wheelchair. But there is a more fundamental point than that:

> Accommodation is a basic human need. The physical and mental health of disabled and able-bodied alike is threatened by homes which are inadequate or lack basic amenities, and the behaviour of all occupants is restrained by dwellings which are structurally unsuited to their physical characteristics; cupboards and sinks of the wrong height, for example, cause discomfort and inconvenience to people who have no impairment other than being too short or too tall.
>
> (Borsay, 1986:68)

Living in a wheelchair increases the likelihood that housing will be unsuitable, for a recent report has estimated that while there are 400 000 wheelchair users in Britain, there are only 42 000 purpose-built or adapted dwellings in the public sector and only 11 000 in the private sector (Ounsted, 1987).

Several studies have pointed to the inadequacies of existing housing and the problems this poses for living with a disability (Buckle, 1971; Finlay, 1978; Borsay, 1986). These deficiencies in provision are likely to cause severe problems for the person with a spinal injury on discharge from hospital. To begin with, he is likely to be discharged to unsuitable accommodation, and this may involve returning to the family home and living in one room where all bodily functions such as eating, sleeping, washing and toileting will take place. It will usually then be a considerable time before more suitable accommodation is provided or the existing house is satisfactorily adapted. This, too, can cause disruption and emotional stress; the person with a spinal injury and his family may not want to move away from existing friends and networks of support, or if adaptations are to be carried out, the disabled person may well have to return to hospital while the work is done.

As we have already suggested, discharge from hospital is likely to be only one step in the disability career, and the person with a spinal injury may wish to move several times throughout his life: to set up his own family, to pursue career opportunities, to retire, and so on.

> This presents a continuing problem, for while the patient may return to an adapted house or be rehoused from hospital, he may well want to change house in the future, especially since spinal cord injuries typically occur in young people who would normally move house several times. A disabled person may have considerable difficulty in finding a suitable house, and there can be time restrictions on further provision of grants for adaptations. Many cannot afford to buy a house and will be dependent on council housing, housing association property, or privately rented property, all of which are in short supply.
>
> (Grundy *et al.*, 1986:41)

For these reasons, people with spinal injuries are likely to have a restricted choice of where to live, to experience considerable delays in obtaining suitable housing and to feel that they lack control of their own lives in this important sphere. These are the themes that will occur in what follows.

HOUSING CIRCUMSTANCES ON DISCHARGE

This, then, raises the issue, already referred to in Chapter 3, concerning where a person may be discharged to, once treatment and rehabilitation at the spinal unit are completed. Table 7.1 gives details of where people were discharged to from hospital. These figures refer to the immediate type of residence, which for some was only an interim measure lasting a short time. Similar figures were arrived at in a study of new injury discharges from the Odstock Spinal Unit 1984–5; 59% returned to their

Table 7.1 Where discharged to from hospital

Discharged to	Number	Percentage
Same residence as before	43	55.8
Different house, same household	8	10.4
Relatives	12	15.6
Friends	2	2.6
Hostel	2	2.6
YDU	5	6.5
Other	5	6.5
	77	100

own homes and 30% were rehoused by the statutory sector or housing associations. The rest purchased more suitable properties. The majority of our people returned to their own homes, or to other accommodation within the community, less than 10% being discharged to some form of residential provision. Perhaps this is just as well if the experience of two people discharged to hostels is anything to go by, for, as one commented:

It just wasn't suitable. I was the youngest person there. I was 18 at the time and the next youngest was 29. And we had all different disabilities— not one other with spinal injuries. There were two blind people, one with muscular dystrophy. Another one had just been put in because his family didn't want him because he was diabetic. I had to go there because Stoke Mandeville discharged me. It was meant to be just for physically handicapped people but there were mentally retarded, and at night times they'd ring the emergency bell and all I'd have all night was the emergency bell going in my ear. There was ex-prisoners and a psychopath who had to be locked up at night. I needed a couple of extra pillows on my bed. They didn't have these. The ones I had on my bed were stained with everything from urine to blood. It was terrible. It was horrible. There was no one there of my own age or with similar disabilities. Some of them were 65 or 70. They'd take all my DHSS for keep and food. I objected to paying all of that out for powdered mash and food you could exist on but it wasn't good. All I had was a room with a bed in. There was a TV lounge where you could watch telly but you had to be in bed by 10, with lights out by 10.30 p.m. so I couldn't watch anything decent. I thought of getting a portable telly but I couldn't have left it because there was some roguish characters there. One of them was selling off the bed linen to local hotels . . . I expect you won't believe me. My social worker said: 'Are you enjoying it?' I said, 'No'.

Similar comments were made by those people who ended up in Young Disabled Units. They complained of being bored, having no privacy, being tied to a routine and generally living out a stultifying existence. One person turned to studying with the Open University as a way of combating his life in an institution:

I first shared a room with three other people and eventually got a room of my own. I was studying with the Open University and I was a lot happier and started coming out of the depression.

Eventually he managed to leave the YDU and now lives with three care attendants in a specially adapted house, but still feels very strongly about his experiences there.

Another person, originally discharged to his parents' home, was offered a job elsewhere and had to move to be near his prospective

employment. The only way he was able to do this was to move to a
nearby Cheshire Home. He described some of the problems that arose:

> The indignities that you have to go through—I'm not saying that all
> Cheshire Homes are the same—but the one I lived in saw its job
> description as providing you with shelter but didn't really accommodate
> your needs. The idea that someone within the home should actually want
> to get involved in self-determination of their life-style was new to them—
> hostile—it was seen as a threat.

He eventually managed to achieve this self-determination, not through
help from the statutory services, but by finding a housing association
willing to provide him with suitable accommodation and getting needs
for care attendants met through the Manpower Services Commission
Community Programme. In recent years more and more disabled people
have struggled and eventually succeeded in living independently
(Shearer, 1983; HCIL, 1986), although the difficulties involved in doing
this should not be minimised.

Not all of those who had lived in residential accommodation were
completely condemnatory. One individual made the following points:

> It wasn't too bad. It's a home where a lot of disabled people are, some old,
> some young. It was sort of mixed. It was supposed to be for young people
> but when I got there I found that about three were young people and the
> rest were old . . . . I had to make myself fit in there. I made myself happy. I
> bought myself a stereo and friends used to come and see me every day
> anyway so I was more or less at home.

He also eventually left the home and set himself up in a flat with an old
school friend. One other person found his local YDU a useful resource
when his marriage broke up, although, again, he eventually left when
he married a nurse he had met while resident there. There are two
points to emphasise here, therefore, concerning residential care. First, it
does have a role to play in some people's lives but it should be available
as a choice, not as the only option. Second, the standard and quality of
this type of provision needs to be substantially improved before it can be
offered as a realistic choice.

HOUSING FROM A CAREER PERSPECTIVE

Most people, however, were discharged back into the community and
we can further utilise the career perspective in looking at changes in
people's housing situations over time, focusing on housing circum-

stances at the time of the accident, on discharge from hospital and at the time of the interview. Table 7.2 looks at house type at those three points in time. From the career perspective, it can be seen that the percentage of people living in houses substantially reduces over time, whereas the proportion living on a single level (in a flat or bungalow) increases. This echoes the words of a Government report, which suggests that 'all that most disabled, even the severely disabled need, is a house or flat on one level' (DHSS, 1974:35). Clearly, however, it takes a considerable time,

Table 7.2 Housing circumstances

House type	At accident	On discharge	At interview
House (%)	68.4	64.5	48.1
Flat (%)	14.5	10.5	23.2
Bungalow (%)	6.6	9.2	26.0
Residential home institution (%)	0.0	9.3	3.0
Other (%)[a]	10.5	6.5	0.0
	100	100	100
Base totals	(76)	(76)	(77)

[a]Including services accommodation, university, etc.

and possibly several moves, before such a situation can be achieved. Not all disabled people, however, necessarily want to live on one level, and again the question of choice is a recurrent theme in looking at the provision of suitable accommodation for those discharged from the spinal unit.

Before considering these issues, we also need to look at changes in tenancy arrangements from a career perspective. From Table 7.3 it is obvious that the two main options open to people discharged from the spinal unit are owner occupation or renting from the local authority, and in both cases, adaptations to the property are likely to prove necessary. What follows, then, is a consideration of some of the issues involved.

Most people who were discharged to the same residence were happy

Table 7.3 Housing tenancy

Tenancy	At accident	On discharge	At interview
Owned (%)	51.3	53.9	63.6
Rented, council (%)	19.7	22.4	24.7
Rented, private (%)	15.8	3.9	3.9
Other (%)	13.2	19.7	7.8
	100	100	100
Base totals	(76)	(76)	(77)

with the decision, though not necessarily with the time it takes to make the house suitable. Thus, one young man whose parents had moved to a more suitable home just after discharge commented:

> It's fabulous, it couldn't be any better . . . we get on well, it's only if you want to be on your own occasionally.

And another said:

> I'm totally contained and independent here.

However, there was a significant minority who were not happy with the blanket assumptions about their returning to their original residence:

> While I was at Stoke I had a row with my family because they tried to mother me and treat me like a baby . . . it was complicated by the social workers because they were trying to get me to go home. Everyone's advice is 'You can't do without your family, you've got to go home', which is a load of crap, they're just saying that because you're disabled.

Another person expressed concern not just about the assumption but at the way the decisions were made:

> A lot of decisions were made behind my back anyway. Me being in bed and my mother going into Dr Silver. Everything was being done through my parents. They come up with the decisions and you just say 'yeah, yeah' and that was it.

One man, who had been living with friends prior to his accident, was discharged to his parents' home, but moved back to live with his friends after 3 months. He described this experience thus:

> It was terrible . . . awful. I was independent before my accident and they were very good to me but they treated me as if I was about 6 years old. I needed my independence and it was also the fact that my parents did everything for me, they wouldn't let me do things. I wanted to do everything for myself and I thought if I stay here too long I'll just fall into the rut of letting them do everything and that will be the end really.

This point is further reinforced by the same man, who, when he went back to living with friends, found:

> I could just about manage. It was a struggle to start with but I had to go through that . . . . Once I got away from my parents I felt I wanted to get back into life and enjoy it.

A major issue, regardless of housing type or tenancy, is that of

getting necessary adaptations to cater for a wheelchair done satisfactorily. There were a few instances where this proceeded well, as with one
man who returned to the same council bungalow he had been living in
prior to injury:

> The council were very good; widened doors, placed in a ramp. The new
> toilet and bathroom were still to be done when I came home but they
> finished very quickly.

Despite the satisfactory experiences of some people, long delays were a
major bone of contention for many others. These delays were not just
inconvenient, but also could cause a great deal of emotional upheaval
and distress in the family due to lack of privacy, unsuitable conditions
making the disabled person more dependent that he would otherwise
be and the problem of overcrowding. The mother of one tetraplegic
spoke of the struggle to obtain the necessary grant:

> I had to fight like hell with the grant people to get the money for the
> conversion and they wouldn't make up their mind how much the
> allowance should be. I had to threaten them with TV, radio and the
> newspapers because I was told there would be a delay of 10–11 months.
> After threatening them, they agreed to do it straight away but you
> shouldn't have to go through that, should you?

Finances weren't the only problem: there was also often a delay in
starting the conversion work. This frequently gave rise to the problem of
where the person with a spinal cord injury should go during the
building work. The mother of one of the people interviewed recounted
her experience thus:

> The problem was where he [the son] should go whilst the extension was
> being built. The builders were knocking down a wall and making a lot of
> dust. The doctor said he should be kept away from the dust but we
> couldn't find anywhere for him to go.

The problem was eventually resolved by his returning to Stoke
Mandeville while the work was carried out, but beds in the spinal unit
are not always available for this purpose. Further, using beds in this way
is very expensive and may prevent people with more urgent medical
needs from gaining admittance.

Another problem with adaptations concerned both their appropriate-
ness and the involvement of the person and his family with the
decision-making process. Thus, the aunt of one of the interviewees
recounted the following experience:

> They took the bath out of the bathroom and put the shower in. They
> moved the toilet and now that's all wrong and they've got to come back

and do it all again. The hand basin is too small. He can't get over it to wash his hands or something like that. He has to go out in the kitchen. The toilet was moved out of the corner into the middle of the bathroom and that's wrong—it's too far away from the wall. They had to move it so that he can transfer from right to left but he can't get the shower chair in properly now. It's inconvenient for his Mum because she can't have a bath now. We asked them just to move the bath but they said 'No', they'd take out the lot. There wasn't any discussion or anything.

Another person, while pleased that Social Services had agreed to install a lift, was angry that it went through the ceiling rather than an external shaft:

I was cross it had to be fitted into the ceiling beause it's going to cost a terrible amount to put it right again .... I wanted a place built on the outside but they wouldn't wear that.

A final theme which recurred concerned the desire of most people that adaptions and equipment should blend in with the rest of the home. As one respondent aptly put it:

I didn't want the house to resemble a hospital. I wanted it to remain my mother's home.

His mother insisted on the same, using economic as well as aesthetic arguments:

The adaptations we had done were as far as possible to make it attractive to an able-bodied person. You pay for the special disabled equipment and why on earth should you make it into a disabled ghetto if you don't need to. It's also cheaper.

The professionals involved, notably social workers and occupational therapists, were sometimes criticised for failing to understand these issues. Many of the problems of delay occurred because of the poor liaison, initially between the hospital and community services, and later between housing and the social services department, with the net result that there was a lack of co-ordination of all the inputs. This resulted in unnecessary delays and subsequent emotional stress for all concerned.

CURRENT HOUSING CIRCUMSTANCES

So far we have utilised the career perspective to show how people's housing circumstances change over time and some of the problems

Table 7.4 Housing circumstances

			Combined figures	
Household composition	*Number*	*Percentage*	*Number*	*Percentage*
Lives alone	15	19.5	(15)	19.5
Paid care attendants CSVs	5	6.5	(5)	6.5
Married	12	15.6	(14)	18.2
Wife and other	2	2.6		
Wife and children <18 years	10	13.0	(15)	19.5
Wife and adult children	5	6.5		
With one parent	5	6.5		
With both parents	7	9.1		
With parent and relative	1	1.3	(22)	28.6
With parents and siblings <18 years	3	3.9		
With parents and siblings >18 years	6	7.8		
With friends	4	5.2	(4)	5.2
Residential establishment	2	2.6	(2)	2.6
	77	100%	77	100%

involved in trying to obtain satisfactory accommodation. We were also concerned to look at people's current housing circumstances and to discover how satisfied or otherwise they might be with them. At the time of interview the variety of home circumstances people were living in are given in Table 7.4. We also asked people about how satisfied they were with their current housing conditions, and Table 7.5 summarises their responses. Major factors influencing people's satisfaction with their housing were physical access, ability to use all of the facilities in the accommodation and adequate heating. Thus, one person who only had an open fire in the living-room said:

I feel the cold a little bit more than I used to and the heating is not really adequate.

Table 7.5 Satisfaction with housing

Level of satisfaction	*Percentage*
Satisfied	71.1
Minor dissatisfaction	15.8
Marked dissatisfaction	5.3
Severe dissatisfaction	7.8
	100 (76)

For this person it was not just a matter of adequacy, however, but also difficulties of lighting and maintaining a coal fire, which he found virtually impossible to do himself, and which thus became an extra task for his wife.

A major element in reported current dissatisfaction concerned the lack of choice over suitable alternative accommodation. This dilemma was starkly put by one man currently living with his family:

> I'm 27 and time's moving on and I suppose really I should think about moving out, but you never really want to because there isn't anywhere to go. I couldn't live in a place of my own because I wouldn't be able to care for myself and then there's only homes to go and I wouldn't like that.

This fear of residential accommodation was described by another who had previously had experience of it:

> I would feel suicidal if I ever had to go back. Maybe as I got old I'd have to, but I want to die in my own home. I don't want someone checking every 15 minutes to see if I am dead.

The issue of choice was not solely about the availability of appropriate accommodation but also about the kind of support available to facilitate independent living. One person who had been discharged to his parental home as an interim measure was experiencing just these kinds of difficulties:

> Social services had been helpful in trying to sort out independent living arrangements but in the meantime I have had difficulty in finding care attendants as an intermediate stage and have had some totally unsuitable people.

At the time of the interview he was using someone from the SIA Care Attendant Scheme but that was only a short-term solution. A further problem that at least one person encountered was that of moving away from the parental home, which had been specially adapted. He wanted to set up home with his fiancee, but was only able to do so if he paid for the adaptations to the new accommodation himself.

While dissatisfaction within the family has been explored in a previous chapter, one person did indicate that there was a direct connection between this and his housing circumstances:

> If we don't meet the mortgage repayments then we're out on the street. It's all right for someone like me. I mean they'd put me in the local hospital or something. But they're not going to take my mum and brother and sister. The Council said to her, 'If you ever get kicked out of your house we could find somewhere for your son but we coulnd't for the rest

of you'. It isn't very nice knowing that you could have a bed that night but your family couldn't.

A few tetraplegics had struggled to live independently through the use of care attendants, and two of these expressed some degree of dissatisfaction. There were two elements to this: recruitment and suitability. As far as recruitment is concerned, one put it thus:

> As far as I can see there doesn't seem to be much support by the organisations in this country to provide anyone to come and look after me at all. I don't know. The situation seemed pretty bad and I spoke to a few people about it and they rather shrugged their shoulders about it.

With regard to suitability, one high tetraplegic had two care attendants, one from the CSV Independent Living Scheme and the other a Danish helper from the Responaut Scheme based at St. Thomas's Hospital, London. However, problems were still encountered:

> I had one CSV that was awful. He left without warning. CSV didn't find a replacement for 3 months so we weren't very happy with that at all. I suppose my needs are difficult. I need someone who can drive and preferably older than my current CSV . . . . I think the eye-opener was that we didn't realise there wasn't a contract and they could just leave . . . . Most CSVs I'm sure are very nice people that wouldn't do that but there is the problem of finding the right helpers.

Not all of those living alone were completely satisfied either. One man put it like this:

> I feel that nobody cares if I live or die. Sometimes I get the impression that I'm entirely alone . . . . I'm not really. I've got relatives and they come and see me . . . a bit pathetic really . . . . You tend to get strange thoughts when you're living alone. It's how you cope with it that counts . . . sometimes I think someone might break in while I'm here and I imagine how I'd cope with it.

Another, while acknowledging loneliness, discussed his perceived difficulties in finding a partner:

> I never envisaged living on my own. I don't like living on my own but circumstances dictate that it's highly unlikely I'll find the ideal situation under which I'd be prepared to give it up. It will take an unusual relationship to do so—that's something I've realised over the last 18 months. Basically I'm fairly independent myself so I'd want someone who is highly independent. My mother hasn't given up hope yet.

The majority of those living alone were happy in this situation. One person, a paraplegic, had lots of support from his family and neighbours, but he recognised that:

I was lucky. I kept the use of my hands and I can manage by myself.

CONCLUSIONS

The major point to arise from this chapter is that the housing needs of people with spinal cord injury are extremely complex and difficulties often arise, necessitating a move to alternative accommodation or the undertaking of major adaptations. Two central themes also emerge from the data: the *time* it takes before suitable accommodation is eventually provided, and the lack of *choice* that is often experienced, in terms of both where to live and who to live with. This issue of choice was also pertinent for the small number who went into residential accommodation, going there usually because there was no other alternative and subsequently finding little or no choice available when wishing to leave. The problems that arise as a consequence can be extremely distressing and disruptive both for the person with the spinal cord injury and for others in the household.

The problems that arise in trying to obtain suitable accommodation are not something that occur only once, immediately upon discharge, but can affect the rest of the person's career in disability. One tetraplegic, who has lived with his parents, in residential accommodation and now independently, poses the problem succinctly (Ford, 1986:7):

My personal living circumstances do not take into account my future needs, changes and choices. The care support I have available to me is an exception, not the rule. What happens if I want to live somewhere else? Social mobility is an option to most people even if they choose not to exercise it. Would it mean starting from scratch all over again? Probably so. What are the implications with regard to continuing support if I wish to live with a partner? Must they accept the role of unpaid carer as the price for a relationship? How do we make such normal living choices part of normal provision?

CHAPTER 8

Significant Living with a Spinal Injury

INTRODUCTION

Throughout this book, we have stressed the importance of meaning for understanding the lives of people with spinal injuries. One of the central ways of giving meaning to life for everyone is through participation in the work process. However, work opportunities are not evenly distributed throughout the population (Lonsdale, 1986) and the question of whether disabled people can have a meaningful life without work has been raised (Warnock, 1978). Work, of course, does not offer only economic benefits for those who have it, but also psychological and social ones, in that it can give a sense of self-esteem to the worker and also provide friendships and a whole range of social contacts which would not otherwise be available.

It is clear that disabled people do not get equal treatment with regard to work as compared with their able-bodied counterparts (Buckle, 1971; Jordan, 1979; Lonsdale and Walker, 1984). This has been confirmed by a recent study, which also suggests:

> ... people with disabilities have always experienced high rates of unemployment.... Not only have they been subject to more unemployment but once in work they are often in low-status, low-paid jobs.
>
> (Lonsdale, 1986:123)

Further, as the Government acknowledges:

> ... once unemployed, disabled people are much more likely to experience much greater problems in regaining work than unemployed people generally.
>
> (MSC, 1982)

Disabled people, then, find it more difficult to get and keep jobs and to obtain the kind of jobs they desire. Specifically with regard to people with a spinal injury, there have been few studies (Goulding, 1976) but a survey of the membership of the Spinal Injuries Association did suggest that:

103

... the figures are suggestive that the unemployment rate amongst SCI cases is well above the national average, and probably also well above the level pertaining nationally amongst those registered as disabled with the Department of Employment.

(Marshall and Oliver, 1979:5)

In this chapter we present our findings about the employment situation of those with a spinal injury, using the career perspective as a framework. Employment circumstances are explored in relation to three chronological points of time: at the time of the injury, on discharge from hospital and at the time of interview. It is important to bear in mind that not all of those we interviewed were available for work; some were in education or retraining programmes and others had retired. The focus of this chapter is, thus, the significance of work or work-related activities and how both these activities and the meanings they have for individuals may change over time.

EMPLOYMENT SITUATION AT THE TIME OF INJURY

At the time of receiving their spinal cord injury the vast majority of those interviewed had been in full- or part-time employment or education (Table 8.1). A small percentage were unemployed, and a further small

Table 8.1   Occupation at time of spinal cord injury

Occupation	Number	Percentage
Education	9	12
Employed	61	79
Unemployed	4	5
Retired	2	3
Other	1	1
	77	100

percentage were retired, which reflected the pattern of age at which the majority of people were injured. We did not ask questions in any detail about the employment situation at the time of the accident but concentrated on discharge and the time of the interview.

EMPLOYMENT SITUATION ON DISCHARGE

Prior to an injury the majority of people not in education were employed and only a few were unemployed. In dramatic contrast, we

Table 8.2 Employment immediately after discharge

Nature of employment	Number[a]	Percentage
Same employer, same job	6	9
Same employer, new job	8	12
New employer, same job	6	9
New employer, new job	7	11
Retraining/study	11	17
Unemployed	28	42
	66	100

[a]Excludes 9 students, 2 retired.

found that after being discharged from hospital almost half were unemployed. Within the group of people who returned to work only 21% returned to the same employer, and less than 18% returned to the same job. For the majority of people who returned to work, there was some change relating to their employment, either within their previous work situation, or when they moved to a new employer or a new type of employment. Eleven people who had been previously in or available for work underwent some retraining or further education, and a small number were involved in retraining while actually in employment. The majority of those returning to employment or retraining did so within a year of being discharged from hospital.

Several factors had an influence on employment status following injury, including the age of the person at the time of injury, the length of time spent in hospital, the level of the lesion and home circumstances. Each of these needs to be considered separately.

The age at which a person was injured appears to be related to subsequent employment. A much lower percentage of those under 25 at the time of injury were unemployed compared with those who had been older. Thus, 26.7% of those who were aged 20–24 were subsequently unemployed, compared with 62.5% of those aged 35–44 years. Also, a much higher percentage of those under 20 at the time of injury went on to retraining or study compared with older age groups. The difficulties of returning to study were faced by the youngest men experiencing spinal injury, and these will be described later. Very few people aged between 25 and 34, and no one who had been 35 or over at the time of injury, had either retrained or returned to study. Issues concerned with unemployment may, therefore, be particularly relevant to those who were older at the time of being injured.

Our conversations with spinally injured men revealed that returning to work was a positive experience for most and that the earlier this was possible the better, although a quick return was not without difficulties. Employers quite often had reservations about employees returning soon after discharge from hospital. Several of those injured felt that this was because the employer had received pessimistic medical reports which had made them less confident about the person being able to cope or do the job. Some of those injured had reservations themselves about returning to work quickly. Several people said that they had felt physically ill after being discharged but had wanted to return to work as soon as possible in spite of this. They feared that they would have become depressed at home, and that advantages in terms of morale and social contacts outweighed the disadvantages of not waiting to regain physical strength. One person said:

> I was pretty low physically and that made me pretty low mentally—the whole thing was a lot of stress but I had to get back.

Mixed feelings, similar to the kinds of uncertainties recalled by people going back to education were expressed about returning to work, as illustrated by the following comments:

> I felt a mixture of apprehension and satisfaction—it was nice to be able to feel you were doing something useful again but I was apprehensive about coping—particularly about not being able to do a full day's work—I would literally run out of steam halfway through a day. And secondly about being acutely aware of my physical limitations and of how other people saw me.

Not everybody shared these feelings. For one or two people, returning to work was not an immediate concern, and they chose not to give priority to doing so.

The length of time a person spent in hospital following his injury was also related to employment following discharge. A higher percentage of those who had a shorter stay in hospital returned to employment compared with those who spent a longer time in hospital. Thus, 53.3% of those who were in hospital for 4–6 months returned to employment, compared with 18.2% of those who were in hospital more than a year. However, 28.6% of those who spent between 10 months and a year in hospital went back to study or retraining, compared with 13.3% of those who had been in hospital between 4 and 6 months.

It is also possible that length of time spent in hospital might be associated with the person's level of lesion. Whereas 61.5% of incomplete paraplegics returned to employment, only 27.3% of complete tetraplegics did so. However, 27.3% of complete tetraplegics underwent retraining or further study, compared with 15.4% of incomplete paraplegics. A higher percentage of tetraplegics compared with paraplegics were unemployed straight after their discharge from hospital.

A number of people moving to a new place of residence after discharge took up some form of employment. One explanation for this is that some people moved to places offering employment possibilities. Some residential accommodation (hostels, for example) offered such opportunities. Several people discussed their experiences of employment undertaken at a new place of residence, and it has to be said that some of these experiences were extremely negative. One person described his experience of residential employment situations where accommodation was linked with a job:

> If you go and live and work there they pay you a pittance. I think it's degrading to be put in that position. OK, it's nice to have the occupation, but people are abused in that situation.

Other people gave examples which illustrate and reinforce this notion of abuse:

> All it was ... well I'd call it slave labour for local firms. For instance, they'd have a bag of say a hundred thousand fuses and you'd have to sort them into packets of ten and put a label in. Or clip shower curtains onto a sales card. Twelve plastic curtain rings. At first I refused to do the work. You know it was such a menial job I'd rather sit in my room all day and listen to records. They'd say you had a choice, but you were choosing the worst of two evils—the great big hessian sacks of curtain rings, or the fuses. You'd work 37½ hours a week. They'd already take all your DHSS money off you for your stay there and you'd end up getting paid £1.20 for a week's work. Oh, and you had to work a week in hand.

However, some individuals responded differently to employment which was ostensibly unacceptable, or situations in which employment did not comprise work of their choice. One person remarked about his work:

> It was a job that I hated but that wasn't the point, that wasn't the point of working. I didn't care what I was doing. The point was to work. You've got to have something to occupy your mind.

Another said:

> They give me nominal payment for a menial job that normally I wouldn't have dreamed of doing but it's something to do. It's something to keep your mind off of things and it gives me enough stimulation to be able to have a conversation in the evenings.

Several other comments suggest that any employment was considered preferable to unemployment. One person, for example, said:

I just could not face the prospect of sitting around doing nothing all day—it was horrible. That's why I ended up working for effectively nothing—less than nothing in terms of the money—but I needed to work. I was in a rut and I had to get out of it.

These points are discussed further later in relation to feelings about unemployment.

A number of people were engaged in highly satisfactory employment, ranging through many different professions. For example, the occupations of some of those we interviewed included a doctor, a teacher, a bank manager, a computer operator, several professional athletes and directors of a variety of business concerns. These people considered their employment to be meaningful and worth-while.

Some people chose to go back to work on a part-time basis initially, as a means of gradual reintroduction into work which might later expand into full-time employment. This was a common sequence of events among those resuming employment soon after discharge from hospital. For some people, phasing in the return to work had to do with regaining strength and physical well-being; for others it was to do with psychological response to returning to work, as described by one man, who said:

I just went in a couple of times a week at first—I had to get used to everything. After 6 weeks I was fine, but you have to get your confidence back—at first I felt so strange—so unsure of myself.

Several people experienced unsatisfactory delays in returning to work. One person who resumed employment 3 years after discharge from hospital outlined several factors which had been prohibitive in his experience. He explained as follows:

I wanted to get back to work but there weren't too many people around me at the time giving me assistance on it.... I was meeting too many negative people.

RETURNING TO EDUCATION

All of those who had been in education at the time of their injury resumed their studies after being discharged from hospital. Over half returned to the educational establishment attended prior to injury. The remainder continued their education but at different institutions. Most of those going back into education did so within the first 6 months of being discharged from hospital, one person had gone back immediately, and everybody had returned within 3 years. One person chose to delay returning to education in order to carefully plan, and avoid unforseen difficulties.

Students intending to resume their studies after injury met with a variety of responses at both institutional and personal levels. At the personal level, some recalled great support and encouragement from individual members of staff. At the institutional level, however, a range of problems were encountered, largely related to access mobility, and also to do with arrangements for care and assistance. Often difficulties were overcome, although this could demand considerable resilience on the part of the spinally injured person, presented sometimes with Hobson's choice:

> Access was appalling. I couldn't go anywhere in my electric wheelchair, I had to be lifted upstairs, but the choice was, 'well if you don't want to come in you can go to another college'.

Others became involved in complicated and drawn-out strategies for making sure that they could continue their education at the establishment of their own choice. One man, for example, resolved not to take a course at a residential college for disabled students, and instead to study at his local technical college, although there were no facilities for disabled students at the time of his application. Members of a local Rotary Club helped to raise money to put in ramps. However, fund raising had taken over 2 years. Several returning students had sought additional funding from charitable organisations and educational trusts, to meet expenses related to their spinal injury which would not be covered by their ordinary grant.

Several education establishments were undoubtedly opposed to admitting disabled students, and confronted intending students with various objections, often of dubious validity. For example, one establishment refused admission on the grounds that the disabled person would be a fire risk. Another institution refused unless the student could be accompanied by his mother and also a care assistant—an arrangement which was predictably impossible. A college which did admit a spinally injured student informed him part-way through his course that he might have to leave if they could not arrange for classes to take place in ground-floor rooms.

For some intending students, it proved impossible to attend the establishment of preference and alternative arrangements had to be found. For example, one Scottish university proved uncompromising, and refused to make provision for a student who wished to return there, having received his injury part-way through a course. The university concerned refused to admit the student on the grounds that they did not have necessary facilities, or the resources to supply them. Eventually he was received by a polytechnic, and although during the research interview he was able to say that 'in the end it all worked out very well indeed', he remembered that 'at the time I found it all a bit harrowing because I had set my heart on going back [to the original University].'

We asked how people had felt about resuming their education after injury, and typically very mixed feelings were recalled. Support from family, friends and colleagues was remembered as important. Many people talked of anxieties they had felt about going back into education, and about how they would initially cope. One person said:

> The hardest bit was going into lectures with a whole crowd of people when you are only just about coming to terms with being disabled yourself. It's difficult.

It was not unusual for people to remark, 'at times I felt that I couldn't go on', or to state that they had doubted the plausibility of their plans, saying, for example, 'I thought I was being silly about it'. One young man, who at the time of injury had been a medical student, recalled a visit from his professor which had taken place at Stoke Mandeville one week after the accident.

> He said to me, 'Don't worry. You'll qualify as a doctor.' And that's what kept me going. It was difficult. At times I thought I couldn't go on. But now, with finals looming near it seems possible.

OCCUPATION AT THE TIME OF INTERVIEW

By the time of interview another six people had retired, compared with the two who had been retired at the time of injury. Forty-one per cent of the sample were currently in full- or part-time employment or education, compared with 90.9% who had been employed or in education at the time of their injury (Table 8.3). At the time of interview,

Table 8.3   Occupation at time of interview

Occupation	Number	Percentage
Full-time employment/education	25	32.5
Part-time, 20+ hours	6	7.8
Part-time, −20 hours	2	2.6
Retired	8	10.4
Not working	36	46.8
	77	100

46.8% were not working, compared with 5.2% who had not been working at the time of injury. Four people who were unemployed after their discharge, and two who had been employed following discharge, were retired by the time of interview. Only one person who had resumed employment after discharge was now unemployed, as opposed to retired. However, of the eleven who had undertaken study or retraining after hospital, only three were employed full-time at interview, and the remainder were unemployed.

Of 46 people who were in employment or education for more than 20 hours a week at the time of interview only a few expressed dissatisfaction (Table 8.4). Where dissatisfaction was expressed it was

Table 8.4 Satisfaction with current employment or education

Level of satisfaction	Number	Percentage
Satisfied	21	67.7
Minor dissatisfaction	6	19.3
Marked dissatisfaction	2	6.5
Severe dissatisfaction	2	6.5
	31	100

Not applicable = 46.

most often minor, and quite often comprised complaints about the physical environment at work and problems with access. Dissatisfaction was expressed where people had accepted a reduction in pay in order to find employment, or were underpaid for what they were doing. Several people were dissatisfied with their level of responsibility at work.

A slightly higher percentage of those aged under 25 years at the time of interview were unemployed, compared with those aged between 25 and 44 years. A very much higher percentage of those aged between 45 and 59 years were unemployed. Of those aged over 60 years, 88.9% were retired. We also found that higher percentages of both complete and incomplete paraplegics were in full-time employment or education than of either complete or incomplete tetraplegics. The incomplete tetraplegic group have the highest percentage of those not working. This is consistent with other trends found for the incomplete tetraplegic group discussed in other chapters.

There was also a link between car ownership and employment status. Of those owning a car which they drove themselves, 52.9% were in full-time employment or education, compared with only 11.8% of those with no car of their own who were in full-time employment or education. There is likely to be a link between car ownership and employment with level of income. Of those people without their own car, 88.2% were also not working. This was summed up by the mother of one person who said:

> He's in a catch-22 situation really. He can't afford a car until he's got a job and he can't get a job until he's got a car.

The overall picture conveyed was of general satisfaction among those in employment, or education, with their work circumstances. One man who said, 'My work is important to me—without it I'd go round the twist' voiced the thoughts of most of those who were employed.

UNEMPLOYMENT

However, the corollary of satisfaction with employment which our research has shown, is dissatisfaction with unemployment, and those who said:

> I would feel on top of the world *if* I had a job.

Of those who were unemployed during the previous 3 months, 72.4% were dissatisfied with their situation: 41.5% were greatly dissatisfied.

The agencies responsible for finding people jobs were not perceived as helpful and Disablement Resettlement Officers (DROs), in particular, came in for disparaging comments. Both the current high rates of unemployment and low expectations on the part of professionals led to the situation where:

> There were a lot of people that weren't looking on the bright side, saying, 'yeah we can sort things out'. It was more like, 'well, hard luck old chum. You're out of work and that's the way it's going to have to be I'm afraid'.

Eventually this man had regained employment through his own efforts:

> I was lucky I came across a couple of executives—management—that decided they were going to give me some help. I got more help from people that shouldn't have been dealing with it than from people who should.

This point about personal contacts proving more helpful than conventional services on 'or not on' offer was made by several people.

Several areas for concern arose in discussion of how those who were unemployed felt about their unemployed role. Many problems of unemployment noted were also mentioned by people who were employed, in thoughts about the possibility of being without work. A major factor in dissatisfaction with being unemployed was boredom, as typically expressed by the following comments:

> I want to work. It would be ridiculous to think that at 26 years old I'll never work again. You know I'm bored to tears.

Many people spoke about how easily they had, or feared they would have, 'got into a rut' without employment. One paraplegic man, expressing concern for spinally injured people without employment or adequate occupation, said:

> People have got to be encouraged to be positive, to get out as much as they can, and not just watch the telly. The favourite one is to get a computer and a telly, sit in front of it all the time, and become a vegetable. You've got to keep busy whatever.

Another person recalled his own similar experience of encroaching lethargy when unemployed, and described the impact which becoming employed had:

> It [going to work] was the best thing I did. I found at home that I was getting very lazy . . . I was getting up at about one in the afternoon. I was getting lazier and lazier . . . I just couldn't be bothered. And then going back to work completely changed me again.

People who were unemployed gave many reasons for feeling dissatisfied:

> You get out of touch with world affairs, out of touch with local affairs and things going on—you lack conversation. Conversation diminishes so much I'm not confident . . . I need to get back into the throes of normality at work. I can't find enough mental stimulation at home.

Another said:

> It's very difficult not to be able to go back to work. All my life I've been an active man . . . but since my accident I've been here at home . . . what can I say?

The importance of keeping busy for unemployed people was often stressed. However, some people clearly were depressed by unemployment and could not foresee any possibility of their situation changing. Several people described repeated unsuccessful attempts to find employment. Despondent feelings about being unemployed could give rise to extremely negative feelings for some. One man's thoughts on the situation illustrate this:

I had 3 years as a gardener [prior to injury]—and there's no way you can do gardening in a wheelchair. So that's 3 years of my life you might as well chuck down the drain. I've got to start again. But from what? What do you do? It's so frustrating. I've got all that knowledge. But I haven't got the body to do it. There's no way I'm going to work indoors on a production line without even a decent wage. It's not that I'm being fussy but there's no way I can sit indoors and stick heads on little dolls—that would drive me crackers. So I'm waiting for something decent to come along but it's hard you know—they think 'disabled—oh yeah, stick them on the production line'.

There were different responses from those who envisaged that they would not return to employment, often, but not always, characterised by a sense of resignation:

I do miss work. It's like somebody cut your hands off. But I have had to accept the fact.

RETIREMENT

Eight people were retired at the time of interview. Three of those retired expressed severe dissatisfaction with their retirement. One of several factors contributing to dissatisfaction was ill-health associated with the spinal cord injury in old age, or associated with early retirement on medical grounds. Often people were dissatisfied because their spinal injury had meant that they were unable to utilise their retirement in the way they had envisaged as able-bodied. There may be some association between ageing and related health factors and satisfaction with retirement. Older people generally expressed more dissatisfaction than did younger, and this reasserts the importance of further research to investigate ageing with spinal cord injury.

CONCLUSIONS

This chapter has highlighted many important issues in the educational and employment experiences of the spinally injured people inter-viewed. To begin with, while all of those in full-time education at the time of their injury returned to study at some point, they often encountered difficulties from the education authorities and in some cases hostility from particular universities or colleges. In addition, while most people were in employment at the time of their injury, less than half were employed after discharge. At the time of the interview, a large percentage were unemployed. Even allowing for current high rates of unemployment nationally, these figures indicate a much higher unemployment rate than the national average and are similar to the findings of a survey of SIA members (Marshall and Oliver, 1979).

Most of those in work expressed satisfaction with their employment, although a significant minority felt that the jobs were unsatisfactory and did not enable personal fulfilment. Those who were employed voiced profound dissatisfaction with this aspect of their lives. Some people were caught in a 'vicious circle': unable to work because they did not have a car, and unable to afford a car because they were not working. We also found that job chances were improved if individuals went back to work as soon as possible after discharge, although a few respondents chose not to return to work immediately, on the grounds that they were not physically or psychologically ready.

Given the important effects that work has on other aspects of people's lives, the high levels of unemployment in our sample, and in the spinally injured population generally, are clearly unacceptable. More needs to be done to enable more people with spinal cord injury to return to work and, hence, to lead more rewarding lives. This would not only improve their quality of life, but also reduce the burden on the taxpayer.

Next we consider income, which is obviously closely related to many of the issues we have been discussing here.

CHAPTER 9

The Financial Consequences of Spinal Injury

INTRODUCTION

As with unemployment, it is true to say that poverty is unequally distributed and in this unequal distribution disabled people get more than their fair share of this poverty (Townsend, 1979). It is generally recognised that the financial consequences of any disability may be deleterious, as a recently published statement shows:

> Even taking account of the available benefits, people with disabilities are still more likely to suffer from poverty than are non-disabled people. Also people who are equally severely disabled can receive widely differing amounts of money according to the cause or origin of their disability, their national insurance contribution record, their age, or their marital status.
> (Disability Alliance, 1987)

The Disablement Income Group (1987) has recently shown how this latter point may operate specifically with regard to spinal injury. A person who is paralysed from the neck, whose injury occurred at work, would get £199.45 per week in benefits; someone who has paid National Insurance contributions but was injured at home would get £91.30; and someone whose injury occurred at birth would get only £75.85. Someone in receipt of legal compensation would probably get in excess of £400 000 for such an injury.

The ways in which these anomalies arise can be seen from the career perspective. Where the accident resulting in the spinal injury occurs can be crucial: if it occurs at work or in the armed forces, then a substantial war or industrial injuries pension will be paid. How it occurs can also be important, for if it can later be proved that the accident occurred as the result of someone else's negligence, then a substantial sum may eventually be paid in settlement. If neither of these conditions applies, then the person concerned will either obtain income through employment—and, as we have shown in the previous chapter, employment is not always easy to keep or find—or be reliant on State benefits, with all their inadequacies (Stowell, 1980). In any case, the cost of living

116

will have risen sharply for both the disabled person and his family (Hyman, 1977; Walker, 1981; Baldwin, 1985). This will affect not just the management of the weekly budget, but also a range of other activities, such as holidays, leisure pursuits, hobbies, eating out, buying clothes, and all the other things which are part of people's standard of living.

FINANCIAL ASPECTS OF THE DISABILITY CAREER

Clearly, then, financial circumstances have a considerable influence on how spinal cord injury will affect both the individual disability career and that of his family. Existing financial resources, whether the person is working or not, the range of disability benefits and the possibility of legal compensation are all factors which can have an influence, as may many others which will be considered in more detail later.

Some people, therefore experienced little or no financial difficulty, for as one person rather openly put it:

I had fairly good financial backing, little rich boy syndrome really . . . so there was no problem with finance.

Another respondent, who had lost his job as a consequence of the accident and consequently suffered a decline in income, said:

I'm feeling the strain more than I thought I would. I took into acount that my cost of living would be higher, but it has been more of a struggle than I thought. I definitely go without things I would like.

The financial circumstances at the time of the accident, as well as how the accident occurred, can have profound effects on the disability career of the individual concerned. At the time of the interviews, we attempted to place our sample in the appropriate socio-economic group. Table 9.1 divided them in this way and also shows that 31.6% of the sample were living on benefits of some sort. Some of these people were the head of the household, while others were living in households where other family members had other sources of income. A further 34.2% of respondents were unable to be classified. Of these, some were receiving benefits but they had additional sources of income, such as work pension or compensation. In addition, it was not always easy to classify people's income because they lived in family or shared household situations, where a variety of joint or co-operative financial arrangements occurred.

In assessing whether people were satisfied with their financial

Table 9.1 Socio-economic group respondent

Group	Number	Percentage
Class I	1	1.3
Class II	15	19.7
Class III	7	9.2
Class IV	2	2.6
Class V	1	1.3
Benefits	24	31.6
Non-classifiable	26	34.2
	76	100

Missing cases = 1.

Table 9.2 Satisfaction with income

Level of satisfaction	Number	Percentage
Satisfied	42	56.0
Minor dissatisfaction	16	21.3
Marked dissatisfaction	11	14.7
Severe dissatisfaction	6	8.0
	75	100

Missing cases = 2.

circumstances or not, around three-quarters said they were, or expressed only minor dissatisfaction (Table 9.2). In an earlier report based on this study, we draw attention to the relationship between work and satisfaction with income:

> ... only 12.5% of those in full-time employment expressed marked or severe dissatisfaction with their financial situation, whereas 36.1% of respondents not working expressed severe or marked dissatisfaction.
>
> (Creek *et al.*, 1987:393)

This dissatisfaction stems not just from the fact that the income derived from work was higher than that from disability benefits, but also because of the psychological and social benefits of working which were discussed in the previous chapter.

From a career perspective, there was a clear relationship between satisfaction with income and length of time since injury, as Table 9.3 shows. Thus, whereas only 30.4% of those injured less than 4 years expressed satisfaction with their current income, the percentage more than doubles for those injured 5 years or more. This suggests that most people with a spinal injury will experience financial difficulties in the period immediately after the accident, but subsequently these difficul-

Table 9.3   Relationship between satisfaction with income and time since injury

	Time (years)			
Level of satisfaction	*0–4*	*5–9*	*10–15*	*Row total*
Satisfied (%)	30.4	63.0	72.0	56.0
Minor dissatisfaction (%)	30.4	18.5	16.0	21.3
Marked/severe dissatisfaction (%)	39.1	18.5	12.0	22.7
	100 (23)	100 (27)	100 (25)	100 (75)

Significance level $= 0.049$.

ties are reduced, either because people obtain work or compensation or because they learn to survive better on a reduced income. In the rest of this chapter, we shall concentrate on those people whose disability career consists of either living on benefits or waiting for compensation.

LIVING ON BENEFITS

Analysis of the qualitative data revealed high levels of anxiety among many respondents who were living on benefits alone. This was a fairly typical comment:

> We just about scrape through each month. Everything's accumulated into one chunk because I live with my mum. If I lived on my own, looking at how much I get, I don't think I could. We find it hard at the end of the month to sort things out, pay the bills and that.

The issue of availability for work figured in the anxiety living on benefits sometimes created. One respondent had an ongoing debate with the DHSS about whether he was fit for work or not, and the DHSS regularly stopped his payments, creating severe financial difficulties. Thus, his mother said:

> We went down to the DHSS and saw the girl and she put down on the report that he was capable of work so he had to see another doctor to get the all clear. Meanwhile he's got no job to go to. We had to go down again and again and he's got no money. They've said it's OK now, that he isn't capable of work and he'll get his money. When he went down to college it stopped again and we all had to go through the channels again. And it shouldn't be because they know that he's disabled and his mum has to pay the rent and they have to eat.

Access to benefits was clearly important and, for some, these were adequate:

> We took all the allowances that were offered us and we were able to live on that as there was no mortgage on the property or rent to pay.

The mother of one of the people interviewed, who was present at the interview, pointed to some of the in-built difficulties in claiming benefits:

> It was difficult to find out what you're entitled to from the DHSS . . . it was all a matter of trial and error . . . you had to know what to ask for and were not advised about other benefits you may be eligible for . . . you've got to ask for it but it's difficult when you don't know what you're eligible for. If you don't know you can't ask.

There were also problems about the basis on which decisions regarding entitlement to particular benefit are made. Thus, one man who had applied for the attendance allowance 2½ years ago, found:

> They refused it to me, but when I applied for it again 6 months ago, when I felt I was less entitled to it, they awarded it to me—such are the vagaries of man.

While the man had been examined by a different doctor on each occasion, his mother felt that there was another, more significant, explanation:

> It was shortly after you'd come back from Stoke Mandeville Hospital and your attitude was that you could do anything, which is part of the training really.

This represents a general problem for disabled people claiming benefits: disabilities have to be emphasised as opposed to abilities, and in order to be certain of getting a particular benefit, the disabled person has to present himself or herself in the worst possible light.

Another aspect of unfairness was the effect that living on welfare benefits could have on the carer's income. The situation varies according to the benefits received by the disabled person. Many carers are unable to go out to work at all, but when they can, most of their earnings will be lost because reductions will be made in the benefits of the person with a spinal cord injury, leaving the household little or no better off. Even the most 'fortunate', those married to people receiving invalidity benefit, feel that this system is extremely unfair. One wife said:

> With Government allowances, I am not allowed to earn more than £45 a week otherwise they then take everything over that off of [her husband's] invalidity benefit. Now that has never changed over, I don't know how many years, but it certainly has never changed since we were married

[1980]. So every time we get a pay rise I have had to cut down my hours and I am now at the stage where I do so little hours that they really can't employ me any more so I am waiting to be put out of a job as soon as they get someone else in.

A final point about the benefits system was that it was sometimes felt to be unfair:

Unfortunately, if you're over 65 when you have an accident you don't get mobility allowance or anything like that.... I think it's unfair but nevertheless, that's the rules.

Certainly it would be difficult to claim that someone over the age of 65 who sustains a complete spinal injury has less or substantially different mobility needs compared with someone under that age.

The impact on the family is a complex issue which is considered in more detail elsewhere, but there is a hidden financial issue which needs to be mentioned here. This is well stated by one respondent, who said:

I don't think my mother is adequately paid for what she does because if I was to live in a hospital, or if I was to live elsewhere, the care I would need would be 24 hours a day, possibly for that to exist would cost in the region of £300 a week. For them to pay her £18 attendance allowance, in total only about £35 a week−I think that is a bit of a cheek for her to give up her life for me.

OBTAINING LEGAL COMPENSATION

Whether or not someone can claim compensation can have significant effects on the individual disability career. Cases usually take years to come to court, and while, for some, interim payments may be made to alleviate immediate financial hardships, others may not know how much they will get or, indeed, whether they will get anything at all, until the case is heard in court. However, compensation is not a possibility for all, and, of the people we interviewed, not all had yet had their claims settled. Only 39.0% of those we interviewed stated that there was any possibility of legal compensation for their injury. Of these, 63.3% (19) had their compensation claim settled at the time of interview. Of those who had some possibility of legal compensation, 59.3% reported that there had been major delays with their claims. The length of time awaiting settlement, or until the completion of the settlement, varied between less than 1 year and 7 years.

Some of these cases were relatively straightforward, but even where

Table 9.4 Legal compensation

Possibility of legal compensation	Number	Percentage
Yes	30	39.0
No	47	61.0
	77	100

Table 9.5

If yes, is it settled?	Number	Percentage
Yes	19	63.3
No	11	36.6
	30	100

Not applicable = 47.

Table 9.6

Major delays with settlement	Number	Percentage
Yes	19	70.3
No	8	29.6
	27	100

Not applicable = 50 (too soon for 3 to say).

they were, time was still an important element. As one person said of his compensation:

> It still took 2 years to get it but it was straightforward .... I found a solicitor that the social worker at Stoke Mandeville Hospital recommended. He was very good, excellent in fact. Everything I wanted to know, he explained it all, as things went along, he was always writing to me or phoning me up. He was always very exact all the time.

Not everyone, even where the outcome was successful, had this kind of experience. One person, whose compensation had taken 4 years to come through, said:

> I was very relieved when it was over. It wasn't just the money element; it was this long-drawn-out process going backwards and forwards about what happened. Today is the first time in 3 years I've talked about it. It's happened so I want to put it behind me and go forward, so it was a relief to get it over with. It was difficult to make future plans, not knowing financially. In the meantime I survived.

Further, a number of people made a similar point about timing of settlement:

> It's when you first have your accident, that's when you want it all sorted out, when you're lying in hospital.

Of eleven people interviewed whose compensation claim had not been settled, five reported major delays in the process. Only one said that no delay had occurred and for three it was too soon to make the question appropriate. Of those cases still in progress, uncertainty is clearly a problem:

> We still don't know if there is any possibility of legal compensation. It's been going on for 2 years now.

And even where a successful outcome is certain, problems still arise:

> It's caused problems because it's been protracted. For things like interim awards, we felt we couldn't go for too many interim awards because of the circumstances. So that was a problem and just all the extra headaches of it all.

The issue of legal compensation had a significant effect on respondents' satisfaction with the financial circumstances. Of those we interviewed who had settled compensation claims, 84.2% reported satisfaction with their financial circumstances, compared with only 9.1% of those with outstanding compensation claims and 55.6% of those who had no possibility of legal compensation. Thus, 54.5% of those awaiting settlement of compensation expressed marked or severe dissatisfaction with their financial position, a much higher percentage than those who had no possibility of legal compensation. A small number of ex-servicemen expressed profound dissatisfaction in not being able to claim compensation for injuries occurring while on duty. It is interesting to note that Parliament has now passed legislation (1987) making such claims possible.

There were a few cases of dissatisfaction even after the claims had been settled. Not everyone received 100% compensation, and one young man, who had broken his neck playing rugby, put it this way:

> The rugby club were insured with minimal cover as being a member of the RFU, a position that has now been changed so that all players are fully covered. I received £8500 compensation which was minimal. Now cover is £100 000 per individual but it's a bit late for me.

There was also one case, a man who had broken his neck diving from a groyne on the beach in the sea, where no compensation had been expected:

> At first I just disregarded it. I spoke to some people and they said there was no chance. I just let it go because I didn't think there was any chance. But then when I was in Stoke Mandeville a firm of solicitors from Manchester came to see me who specialise in spinal injury compensation, you know, accidents. They spoke to me and compensation resulted from that.... I don't know why they came, I think they were just in the hospital that day. I got compensation of £20 000 which I was amazed about. I wasn't expecting anything.

One individual found that the possibility of compensation had adversely affected his relationship with his family:

> My family were obsessed with the money and were convinced that my girlfriend was after the money she thought I'd get. I used to think, 'it can't be true, they can't be like that'. It turned out that all they were interested in was the money.

A few respondents, in receipt of large compensation payments, expressed ambivalence rather than satisfaction or dissatisfaction. One said:

> Having big compensation is a problem. How do you motivate yourself then?

While most people who were able to claim compensation end up being satisfied with the outcome, the process of claiming causes difficulties for many individuals and their families. There is also the problem that this system poses for the rehabilitation process, which is well summarised in a recent review of the disability income system:

> Arguments about the effects of tort* on incentives to rehabilitation revolve around the problem of delay and the effect of lump sum payments. Since the amount of damages will be related to the extent of residual disability, it is argued that incentives to undertake rehabilitation are adversely affected while a tort claim is pending. Given that the more serious the injuries the longer the claim process, this disincentive to rehabilitation, if it exists, is most damaging where an active programme of rehabilitation is most needed. As a general rule the maximum benefit can only be obtained from rehabilitation, from the medical point of view, if it is undertaken without undue delay and before preventable impairment develops. Thus the delays before settlement may well lead to an unnecessarily high level of

---

*Tort is a legal term which refers to the need to prove that someone else was at fault (negligent) and thus caused the injury to occur.

disability which cannot subsequently be overcome. Whether tort does act as a disincentive depends of course on the individual's reaction to the situation in which he finds himself, but as a theoretical position the case against tort on this point is a convincing one.

The actual payment of a lump sum is, on the other hand, considered likely to promote rehabilitation, since, once made, it cannot be taken back and a programme of recovery which produces a reduction of the effects of disability and of the possible income loss becomes highly desirable. This has been used as an argument against changing from lump sum settlements to periodic payments which might be adjusted downward if there was unexpected improvement. In spite of the possible benefits of the lump sum method of payment, it must on the whole be concluded that the tort system is not favourable to rehabilitation, since it places the injured person in the position that he must choose in the first instance between a greater degree of recovery which may prove to be temporary and a higher level of compensation. Thus it becomes one more element in the tort lottery.

(Brown, 1984:337–8)

Clearly, then, the need to prove that someone else was to blame for the injury can adversely affect the rehabilitation process of the injured person. Not only that, but, as we have seen, the delays and uncertainties that occur as a consequence of the legal process may cause severe financial hardship and create profound personal and family anxieties.

A number of solutions have been posed to this clearly anomalous situation, including a national disability income and a no-fault compensation system. This is not the place to discuss the advantages and disadvantages of these proposed solutions, but we need to point out that, from our data, the current system is clearly unsatisfactory and causes much hardship and human misery, even when the final outcome is successful.

CONCLUSIONS

There are three major ways in which individuals with spinal injuries can obtain an income: through work, through the disability benefits system and through claiming compensation through the courts. While gaining income through employment was clearly the most satisfactory way of being in a sound financial situation, nearly half of our sample were not working at the time of the interview. Compensation usually produced a more than satisfactory financial situation if the claim was successful, but much hardship and distress was caused in pursuit of it. Those whose financial circumstances were most unsatisfactory, were those whose sole or main income was benefits.

Living a career in disability may be difficult enough, given the medical, personal, interpersonal, social and environmental problems that the person with spinal cord injury may have to face. But all or any of these problems are compounded by the economic constraints that many of the people we interviewed face, and while we would not want to argue that money can ever adequately compensate for becoming spinally injured, it can add choice and meaning and significantly improve the overall quality of life. For this reason, people with a spinal injury need a coherent and equitable system to meet their financial needs rather than the present system, which operates like a giant one-armed bandit, whereby what you get out of the system depends upon a whole series of chance factors and is unrelated to individual needs.

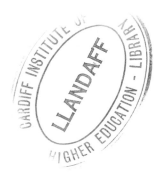

CHAPTER 10

Conclusions: What Kind of Life?

INTRODUCTION

Since the end of World War II, the progress of medical science and rehabilitation has literally transformed the lives of many thousands of paraplegics and tetraplegics, who previously would, quite simply, have died. However, the central issue for the late twentieth century is not whether people with a spinal injury can be kept alive, but what kind of life they can expect. This issue of the quality of life is of central importance, not just to those already spinally injured, but also to the 400 or so who will continue to be so injured every year into the forseeable future. Therefore, in order to improve existing services and plan and deliver future ones, it is important to have a clear idea about what is wrong with the existing pattern of provision. To paraphrase an often-quoted saying, 'we can't possibly know where we are going unless we know where we have been'. It is particularly important to have an understanding of the defects in services and provision from the point of view of those who use, and in many cases are reliant upon, them. As far as we are aware, ours is the first study which attempts to provide this point of view, at least in respect of people with spinal injuries.

Before proceeding to look at some of the implications of our study, it is necessary to point out some of its limitations. First, our study was based on people discharged from the NSIC, Stoke Mandeville Hospital, only. This was the first and remains the largest of all the Units and consequently has the largest catchment area. Second, it was a retrospective study and the Unit moved to a brand new building in 1982. Third, our study was confined to men for methodological reasons, although we await with interest the publication from the Women's Group of the Spinal Injuries Association of their study of the experience of women with spinal injuries.

Despite these limitations, we believe that our study offers a sufficiently representative view of the disability careers of people with spinal injuries for us to make a number of suggestions as to how services to this group of people might be improved in the future. We have come to this belief not simply because of our own personal contacts with individuals with spinal injuries, but also on the basis of the feedback we have had from the publication of our original report (Creek *et al.*, 1987) and from the three conferences we have held to present our findings.

THE SPINAL INJURIES SERVICE—FROM ACCIDENT TO GRAVE?

In an ideal world there would perhaps be no need for a specialist spinal injuries service to exist, and all those so injured could be treated and rehabilitated in the hospital nearest to their own homes. However, it is clear that general hospitals do not possess the expertise to treat the newly injured, to provide adequate rehabilitation programmes or to deal with the medical and other complications that may arise for the rest of the disability career. Further, many of those treated in these hospitals at present may develop unnecessary complications which can necessitate extra time spent in a specialist unit, or may experience the constant breaking down of pressure sores contracted in the general hospital. There is no doubt that the vast majority of those we interviewed would prefer all their treatment, of whatever kind, to be provided by the spinal unit, and this is a view strongly supported by the leading consumer group, the Spinal Injuries Association.

Some people may, at present, have access to the service from accident to grave, but not everyone who breaks his spine reaches a specialist unit, and many of those who do may never return after discharge. The Unit at Stoke Mandeville currently estimates that it has 6000 ex-patients and less than half of these are seen on a regular basis or systematically followed up. This mirrors our own findings, where only half of those we interviewed had had further contact with the Unit. There are obviously resource implications from such a service but it is difficult to estimate what these might be, for no central record of the numbers of people with a spinal injury are kept. Clearly, such records are the basis on which an accident to grave service could be planned and provided and thus are urgently needed. Further, the failure to provide such a service undoubtedly results in unnecessary suffering and misery and also itself uses up resources through the development of medical complications, the blocking of scarce beds, and so on.

BETTER CO-ORDINATION OF EXISTING SERVICES

A major problem that many of those we interviewed experienced was the poor co-ordination of services, particularly on discharge from the spinal unit. As we have already intimated, this may partly be a problem of the size of the catchment area of Stoke Mandeville, but distance alone cannot account for the problems experienced when agency boundaries are crossed. In addition, often the services that were provided after discharge did not match what people felt they needed or, indeed, what they were entitled to. Finally, services were fragmented and subject to much local variation, often depending on the place of residence or the commitment and competence of the individual professionals concerned.

More specifically, both health and social service professionals were criticised for their lack of knowledge of spinal injury and for the inflexibility and inappropriateness of the services they sometimes offered. Aids and equipment were in short supply and therefore often difficult to obtain, and there was usually no ongoing or long-term support for the disabled person or his family.

Even allowing for the distances involved, there is an urgent need for better mechanisms for co-ordinating services between the Spinal Unit and the local authorities it serves, perhaps through the appointment of a home liaison officer, who would be the central point of contact and who could visit each local authority to facilitate transfer. A closer involvement of people with spinal injuries is also required if the gap between what people feel they need and what services are able or willing to provide is to be significantly reduced. The training of all professionals also needs to be considerably improved, and again this can only be done by using the knowledge and expertise available within the spinal injury service and by fully utilising the experience of those with a spinal injury. While these suggestions will obviously have cost implications, a great deal can be done by changing attitudes and practices among professionals. Certainly, services which were most likely to be perceived positively were those which were delivered 'in partnership'.

CHANGES AT NSIC

While, on the whole, people were very appreciative of the treatment and care they received in the Unit, there were four criticisms that need to be reiterated here. First, many people were critical about the manner in which they were told about their injury, feeling that it was spelt out too bluntly or perhaps before they were ready. Others, on the other hand, appreciated the honesty, and some of those who had initially been upset or angry felt, in retrospect, that it was perhaps the best way. Second, the rehabilitation programme was felt to be too physicalist and inflexible, with everyone, regardless of age, different needs or goals, being processed on the same conveyor belt. Third, there was little attention paid to the emotional needs of the individuals concerned and they were provided with little or no help or information with regard to personal matters such as sexuality. Fourth, the lack of any systematic system for monitoring and providing people with check-ups meant that many people may have had no further contact with the Unit after initial discharge, and this may have important subsequent effects on their disability career.

Given the strength of feeling that we found, often many years later, the whole issue of when and how to tell someone the true extent and nature of their injury needs to be reviewed. As all individuals are different, individual strategies may need to be operated: some may be told, as now, as early as possible and in a one-to-one situation with the consultant; others may be told with other close family members present; and still others may be told in the presence of other professionals or allowed to find out informally through contact with other people with spinal injuries. It should be relatively simple to tailor the rehabilitation programme to the needs of individuals, and working towards the patient's own self-defined goals should help to make the programme less physicalist. The Unit has already recognised the need to develop services to meet the emotional needs of patients with the appointment of a clinical psychologist and we would hope to see a peer counselling scheme introduced as well, as such schemes have proved successful in the United States. A computerised record system should make it easier to provide ongoing monitoring for all ex-patients. This could also prove to be cost effective in significantly reducing the numbers of long-term readmissions, for, by identifying problems in their early stages, beds could be freed for the newly injured.

BRINGING THE FAMILY IN

The existence or otherwise of a supportive family can have a profound impact on the outcome of the disability career. Both within the Spinal Unit and subsequently after discharge, families—and primary carers in particular—are often left with little or no support or even acknowledge-ment of the vital role they perform. The major focus is on the person with the spinal injury, and family members often felt that they were provided with little or no emotional support themselves while their relative was in hospital. Further, they felt excluded from many of the tasks carried out by nursing staff on the wards when after discharge they would be expected to carry out these tasks alone and unsupported. They also felt excluded from choice about whether the injured person should return to the family or not; it was simply assumed by all the professionals concerned that the person should be returned to the family, even when the person had not been living in the family home prior to discharge. Once back in the community, this situation was reproduced, with the added problem that little or no long-term support was provided for family members, and few facilities such as respite care existed.

It is in no one's interest to neglect this situation, for it can precipitate family break-up and place more pressure on statutory services, both hospital and community. There has been some attempt at the Unit to set up family groups to support relatives, but a thorough review of the role of the family and the provision of appropriate services for them needs to take place. Similarly, in the community, the current initiatives to provide support for carers need to be built upon and made widely available to the carers of those with a spinal injury, and these services should be available on an ongoing basis and not simply when the family reaches crisis point. Whatever services are provided, a spinal injury can have a shattering impact on the family, but some of the emotional distress and suffering can be alleviated through the provision of appropriate services.

LIFE IS FOR LIVING

Most people with a spinal injury were able to continue with their lives, leisure pursuits and social contacts, and although changes in these activities occurred over time, a happy and fulfilling life was possible. However, there were a number of restrictions placed on these aspects of people's lives, including physical access to buildings, the inaccessibility of public transport, the problems of obtaining the right kind (particularly electric) of wheelchair and sometimes the cost of running a car. In terms of personal relations, people sometimes felt that the wheelchair was a barrier to forming relationships, and dependence on their families for high-lesion tetraplegics often made this difficult.

Personal relationships are not something in which it is necessarily appropriate to intervene in terms of recommendations for policy or practice. However, we have no doubt that the social lives of people with spinal injuries could be significantly improved with improvements to the physical environment, including buildings and transport systems. In addition, the provision of the right wheelchairs and adequate financial assistance to purchase cars could open up more opportunities for leisure and add to the quality of their social lives for this group of people.

A PLACE TO LIVE

As most of the housing stock in the United Kingdom, in both the public and the private sectors, is unsuitable for people in wheelchairs, sudden disability through spinal cord injury can create severe difficulties in this area. Thus, often there is little suitable existing housing into which someone can move on discharge from hospital, and the only option may be to adapt existing accommodation, if this is possible. Even if adapting the existing house is possible, the various agencies concerned are usually unable to do this in time for the person's return from hospital, causing further difficulties for the person and his family. These problems are compounded if a person wishes to move at various stages in his disability career. Finally, there are few flexible care attendant schemes available to facilitate choices not just about where to live, but also who to live with, and the quality of residential provision is so poor that few people choose it voluntarily but enter it only as a last resort.

In the long term, the only way forward is to increase the stock of 'wheelchair' and 'mobility' housing in both sectors, as advocated by the Department of the Environment. In the short term, the Spinal Unit, the Social Services and the Housing Departments need to significantly improve their communication and liaison procedures in order that unsuitable housing can be made suitable much more quickly. Improved residential facilities and flexible support services in the community would obviously widen the choices available, but we should point out that we do not believe that residential care is necessary for anyone with a spinal injury, no matter how disabled he or she is, unless this option is freely chosen from a range of acceptable alternatives.

A GOOD AND USEFUL LIFE

Work and education are as important to people with a spinal injury as they are to everyone else and not simply because of the financial rewards they can bring. Spinal injury can clearly have a drastic effect on the work situation, for less than half of the people we interviewed were employed at the time of the interview. On the other hand, all of those who wished to return to education were able to do so, albeit with various difficulties of one kind or another. The issue of retirement is a complex one, which we are currently studying further as part of a broader research project looking at ageing and spinal injury.

A more positive approach to the issue of work for people with a spinal injury is obviously needed, and we hope that the statutory agencies charged with responsibility in this area, particularly the Manpower Services Commission, will take note. It is our impression that those with a spinal injury feel that they have a right to education if they so choose, and many educational institutions support this rights-based approach through their own policy statements and admissions procedures. A similar enlightened approach needs to be operated in terms of work, and this could be achieved by the MSC adopting an enforcement rather than persuasionist approach to the Disabled Persons (Employment) Act 1944.

MONEY MAKES A DIFFERENCE

No amount of money can compensate for disability arising from spinal cord injury, but for those living on benefits, the money available will often not even buy the basic necessities of life. Attendance allowance and mobility allowance, provided to meet specific needs, are often absorbed in the family budget in the struggle for survival. Compensation will, in the long run, provide more satisfactory financial remuneration, but it usually takes a long time to get, and can adversely affect the rehabilitation process and cause much interim hardship and suffering. Income through work, usually though not always, provides the most satisfactory mechanism for remuneration because of its social as well as economic aspects, but even those in well-paid jobs do not fare as well as do their able-bodied counterparts, because of the extra costs of living with a disability.

If people with a spinal injury are to have the financial resources to live a full and happy life, then a positive approach to employment of this group needs to be adopted, supplemented by an adequate system of benefits, both to meet the extra costs of disability for those in work and to provide an adequate income for those who are not. Were such a system in existence, it is an open question as to whether we would need a compensation system as well. Our own view is that the compensation system is based on chance factors related to how the accident occurred rather than geared to meet needs, and is therefore unnecessarily divisive. However, we are pessimistic about the implementation of such an approach in the forseeable future, and we fear that the changes in the social security system will, in fact, create further financial difficulties for those already injured and place a severe financial burden on all those yet to be injured.

SOCIAL ADJUSTMENT – A CONTINUOUS AND RECIPROCAL PROCESS

We have been concerned to locate our analysis within a framework which did not simply focus on medical aspects of spinal injury or on the psychological factors after injury. That is not to say that we have sought to deny the importance of these factors for some people at some points in their disability careers, but rather to suggest that they have to be considered alongside a range of other personal, social and material factors.

In order to do this, we have suggested that disability can only be understood as a relationship between individual impairment and its social consequences. To facilitate this, we have utilised the concept of social adjustment as a way of understanding this relationship. This, then, implies that satisfactory social adjustment is not just dependent upon a range of personal and psychological processes that an individual must go through, but also on the way that external factors impinge on this relationship. For this reason, in this concluding chapter, we have concentrated on the ways in which some of these external factors can be improved in order that satisfactory social adjustment can be achieved.

Furthermore, social adjustment is not a once and for all thing: it may change over time as an individual's needs and wishes change and also as the circumstances in which he finds himself change. Thus, we have also made use of the idea of the disability career in order to give a temporal coherence to our work, and it is clear that time is a significant factor in social adjustment within the disability career. From our findings, it can take at least 9 years for individuals to become socially adjusted in terms of both personal responses and external circum-stances. A satisfactory service to people with spinal injuries must take account of this and provide ongoing and comprehensive support both in hospital and in the community.

Finally, we are anxious that our work should not become another inflexible conceptual framework on which to base service provision and treatment, but rather a way of understanding the disability relationship. Thus, we also used the concepts of significant life events and meaning to demonstrate that, within the broad processes of social adjustment to the disability career, the ways individuals responded to their injuries were often highly personal: individuals with the same level of lesion and living in similar material circumstances might feel and respond very differently to spinal injury as a significant event in their lives. Thus, an effective spinal injury service needs to be organised to provide ongoing and comprehensive support, but it also must be sufficiently flexible to meet the needs and wishes of people with spinal injuries as they themselves define them.

LIFE EXPECTANCY OR EXPECTATION OF LIFE?

We hope, in this book, we have shown that the recent history of spinal injury has been a triumphant one in terms of keeping people alive, and the crucial issue we now have to address concerns the quality of those lives. We would not wish our work to be seen as simply an indictment of the failures of the services that have been established for people with spinal injuries but, rather, a constructive attempt to identify the defects and weaknesses of these services from the point of view of those who use them, and to suggest ways in which these services could be improved. In so doing, we have relied on the words of those people with spinal injuries who were often able to identify a problem or articulate an issue so much more eloquently than us. It is, therefore, fitting that we end with two such statements, which say things so succinctly. One man, on being asked what it was like being discharged from Stoke Mandeville, responded:

It was like walking into darkness.

And another, when asked about his current situation, stated:

I think my life could be better than this, it should be.

References

ACC (1985). *Strategies for Community Care* (London, Association of County Councils)

Audit Commission (1986). *Making a Reality of Community Care* (London, HMSO)

Baldwin, S. (1977). *Disabled Children—Counting the Costs* (London, The Disability Alliance)

Baldwin, S. (1985). *The Costs of Caring* (London, Routledge and Kegan Paul)

Barclay Committee (1982). *Social Workers, their Role and Tasks* (London, NCVO/NISW)

Barker, J. and Bury, M. (1978). 'Mobility and the elderly: a community challenge'. In Carver, V. and Liddiard, P. (Eds.), *An Ageing Population* (London, Hodder and Stoughton)

BCODP (1987). *Comment on the Report of the Audit Commission—Making a Reality of Community Care* (British Council of Organisations of Disabled People)

Blaxter, M. (1980). *The Meaning of Disability* (London, Heinemann)

Borsay, A. (1983). 'Are occupational therapists cinderellas?' *Social Policy and Administration*, **17** (2), 130–141

Borsay, A. (1986). *Disabled People in the Community: A Study of Housing, Health and Welfare Services* (London, NCVO/Bedford Square Press)

Bradshaw, J., Glendinning, C. and Baldwin, S. (1977). 'Services that miss their mark and leave families in need'. *Health and Social Services Journal* April, 664–65

Bray, G. P. (1977). 'Reactive patterns in families of the severely disabled'. *Rehabilitation Counselling Bulletin*, **20**, 236–239

Bray, G. P. (1978). 'Rehabilitation of spinal cord injured: a family approach'. *Journal of Applied Rehabilitation Counselling*, **9**, 70–78

Briggs, A. and Oliver, J. (1984). *Caring: The Experience of Looking after Disabled and Elderly Relatives* (London, Routledge and Kegan Paul)

Brown, G. and Harris, T. (1979). *Social Origins of Depression* (London, Tavistock)

Brown, J. (1984). *The Disability Income System* (London, PSI)

Buchanan, J. M. and Chamberlain, M. A. (1978). *Survey of the Mobility of the Disabled in an Urban Environment* (London, RADAR)

Buckle, J. (1971). *Work and Housing of Impaired People in Great Britain* (London, HMSO)

Carver, V. (1982). 'The individual behind the statistics'. Unit 3 in *The Handicapped Person in the Community (Block 1)* (Milton Keynes, Open University Press)

CCETSW (1974). *People with Handicaps Need Better Trained Workers* (London, Central Council for Education and Training in Social Work)

Cook, D. W. (1976). 'Psychological aspects of spinal cord injury'. *Rehabilitation Counselling Bulletin*, **19**, 535–543

Creek, G., Moore, M., Oliver, M., Salisbury, V., Silver, J. and Zarb, G. (1987). *Personal and Social Implications of Spinal Cord Injury: A Retrospective Study* (London, Thames Polytechnic)

Davis, K. (1981). '28–38 Grove Road: accommodation and care in a community setting'. In Brechin A., Liddiard, P. and Swain, J. (Eds.), *Handicap in a Social World* (London, Hodder and Stoughton)

Denby, E., Taylor, P. and Peach, M. (1978). *Guides 1–5* (London, Islington Access Project)

DeVivo, M. J. and Fine, P. R. (1985). 'Spinal cord injury: its short-term impact on marital status'. *Archives of Physical Medicine and Rehabilitation*, **66**, 501–504

DHSS (1968). *Report of the Committee on Local Authority and Allied Social Services* (The Seebohm Report) (London, HMSO)

DHSS (1974). *Aids to Households: England* (London, HMSO)

DHSS (1976). *Priorities for Health and Personal Social Services in England: A Consultative Document* (London, HMSO)

DHSS (1978). *Social Services Teams: The Practitioners View* (Stevenson, O. and Parsloe, P., Eds.) (London, HMSO)

DHSS (1981). *Care in Action: A Handbook of Policies and Priorities for the Health and Personal Social Services in England* (London, HMSO)

DHSS (1986). *Review of Artificial Limb and Appliance Centre Services* (The McColl Report) (London, HMSO)

Disability Alliance (1987). *Poverty and Disability: Breaking the Link* (London, Disability Alliance)

Disablement Income Group (1987). *DIG's National Disability Income* (London, Disablement Income Group)

Dohrenwend, B. and Dohrenwend, B. (Eds.) (1974). *Stressful Life Events: Their Nature and Effects* (New York, Wiley)

Finkelstein, V. (1980). *Attitudes and Disabled People: Issues for Discussion* (New York, World Rehabilitation Fund)

Finlay, B. (1978). *Housing and Disability: A Report on the Housing Needs of Physically Handicapped People in Rochdale* (Rochdale Voluntary Action)

Ford, C. (1986). 'Collaboration: a personal experience of social work in application' (Paper presented at BASW–BCODP Conference–*Disabled People and Social Workers, Changing Philosophy, Changing Practice*)

Forder, A., Reti, T. and Silver, J. (1974). 'Communication in the Health Service: a case study of the rehabilitation of paraplegic patients'. In Boswell D. and Wingrove J. (Eds.), *The Handicapped Person in the Community* (London, Tavistock)

Fox, A. M. (1974). *They Get This Training but They Don't Know How You Feel* (London, RADAR)

GLAD (1986). *Consumer Study of Transport Handicap* (London, Greater London Association for Disabled People)

Glendinning, C. (1986). *A Single Door: Social Work with the Families of Disabled Children* (London, Allen & Unwin)

Goffman, E. (1961). *Asylums* (New York, Doubleday)

Goffman, E. (1963). *Stigma: Some Notes on the Management of Spoiled Identity* (Englewood Cliffs, N.J., Prentice-Hall)

Goodman, S. (1986). *Spirit of Stoke Mandeville: The Story of Sir Ludwig Guttmann* (London, Collins)

Goulding, C. (1976). *Employment of Tetraplegics* (Sussex, National Fund for Research into Crippling Diseases)

Grundy, D., Russell J. and Swain A. (1986). 'ABC of spinal cord injury'. *British Medical Journal*, special edition

Guttmann, L. (1964). 'The married life of paraplegics and tetraplegics'. *Paraplegia*, 2

Guttmann, L. (1976a). 'Significance of sport in rehabilitation of spinal paraplegics and tetraplegics'. *Journal of American Medical Association*, 236, 1975–1977

Guttmann, L. (1976b). *Spinal Cord Injuries: Comprehensive Management and Research*, 2nd edn (Oxford, Blackwell)

Hasler, F. and Oliver, M. (1982). *Social Work in a Self-Help Group: A Case Study of the Spinal Injuries Association* (London, Spinal Injuries Association)

HCIL (1986). *Project 81: One Step On* (Hampshire Centre for Independent Living)

Hoad, A. (1986). *The Impact of Transport on the Quality of Life and Lifestyles of Young People with Physical Disabilities* (London, London School of Hygiene and Tropical Medicine)

Howe, D. (1980). 'Divisions of labour in the area teams of Social Services departments'. *Social Policy and Administration*, 14(2), 135–142

Hyman, M. (1977). *The Extra Costs of Disabled Living: A Case History Study* (National Fund for Research into Crippling Diseases)

Jordan, D. (1979). *A New Employment Programme Wanted for Disabled People* (Disability Alliance)

Jowett, S. (1982). *Young Disabled People: Their Further Education Training and Employment* (Windsor, NFER)

Keeble, U. (1979). *Aids and Adaptations* (London, Bedford Square Press)

Kerr, W. and Thompson, M. (1972). 'Acceptance of disability of sudden onset in paraplegia'. *International Journal of Paraplegia*, 10, 94–102

Lonsdale, S. (1986). *Work and Inequality* (London, Longman)

Lonsdale, S. and Walker, A. (1984). *A Right to Work* (London, Disability Alliance)

Marshall, T. and Oliver, M. (1979). *Work and Disability: An Employment Survey of Paraplegics and Tetraplegics* (London, Spinal Injuries Association)

Mechanic, D. (1962). *Students Under Stress* (New York, Free Press)

Miller, E. and Gwynne, G. (1971). *A Life Apart* (London, Tavistock)

Manpower Services Commission (1982). *Review of Assistance for Disabled People* (London, MSC)

Mulroy, B. (1985). 'General practitioner and long-term care of patients with a spinal injury'. *British Medical Journal*, 291, 575–577

Murray, W. and Thompson, A. (1967). *Paraplegia at Home: A Pilot Survey of the Management and Rehabilitation of Paraplegic Patients in Scotland* (Edinburgh, Livingstone)

Oliver, J. (1984). 'The caring wife'. In Finch, J. and Groves, D. (Eds.), *A Labour of Love: Women, Work and Caring* (London, Routledge and Kegan Paul)

Oliver, M. (1981). 'Disability, adjustment and family life: some theoretical considerations'. In Brechin, A., Liddiard, P. and Swain, J. (Eds.), *Handicap in a Social World* (London, Hodder and Stoughton)

Oliver, M. (1983). *Social Work with Disabled People* (Basingstoke, Macmillan)

Ounsted, D. (1987). *Wheelchairs No Handicap in Housing* (National Federation of Housing Associations)

Owens, P. (1987). *Community Care and Severe Physical Disability* (London, Bedford Square Press/NCVO)

RCS (1984). *Report of the Working Party on Spinal Injuries Units* (Royal College of Surgeons of England)

Richards, B. (1975). 'An evaluation of home care after spinal cord injury'. *Paraplegia*, **12**, 263–267

Richards, B. (1982). 'A social and psychological study of 166 spinal cord injured patients from Queensland'. *Paraplegia*, **20**, 90–96

Rogers, M. A. (1978). *Paraplegia: A Handbook of Practical Care and Advice* (London, Faber)

Rowan, P. (1979). *What Sort of Life?* (Windsor, NFER)

Safilios-Rothschild, C. (1970). *The Sociology and Social Psychology of Disability and Rehabilitation* (New York, Random House)

Schulz, R. and Decker, S. (1985). 'Long-term adjustment to physical disability: The role of social support, perceived control and self-blame'. *Journal of Personality and Social Psychology*, **48**, 5

Shearer, A. (1983). *Living Independently* (London, CEH/Kings Fund)

Siller, J. (1969). 'Psychological situation of the disabled with spinal cord injury'. *Rehabilitation Literature*, **30**, 290–296

Silver, R. and Wortman, C. (1980). 'Coping with undesirable life events'. In Gerber, J. and Seligman, M. (Eds.), *Human Helplessness, Theory and Applications* (London, Academic Press)

Silver, J., Oliver, M. and Salisbury, V. (1984). *A Retrospective Study of Spinal Cord Injured People. A Pilot Study* (unpublished)

Stowell, R. (1980). *Disabled People on Supplementary Benefit* (London, DIG)

Townsend, P. (1979). *Poverty in the United Kingdom* (Harmondsworth, Penguin)

Trieschmann, R. (1980). *Spinal Cord Injuries* (Oxford, Pergamon)

UPIAS (1976). *Fundamental Principles of Disability* (London, Union of the Physically Impaired Against Segregation)

Vargo, F. A. and Stewin, L. L. (1984). 'Spousal adaptation to disability: ramifications and implications for counselling'. *International Journal for the Advancement of Counselling*, **7**, 253–260

Walker, A. (1981). Disability and income. In Walker, A. and Townsend, P. (Eds.), *Disability in Britain: A Manifest of Rights* (Oxford, Robertson)

Warnock Report (1978). *Special Educational Needs: Report of the Committee of Enquiry into the Education of Handicapped Children and Young People*. Cmnd. 7212 (London, HMSO)

Weller, D. and Miller, P. (1977). 'Emotional reactions of patient, family and staff in the acute care period of spinal cord injury'. *Social Work in Health Care*, **3**

Wilding, P. (1982). *Professional Power and Social Welfare* (London, Routledge and Kegan Paul)

Index

Page numbers in italics indicate that relevant tables are included.